BALANCE YOUR LIFE, BALANCE THE SCALE

BALANCE YOUR LIFE, BALANCE THE SCALE

DITCH DIETING, AMP UP
YOUR ENERGY, FEEL AMAZING, AND
RELEASE THE WEIGHT

JENNIFER TUMA-YOUNG

HarperOne
An Imprint of HarperCollinsPublishers

HarperOne

This book is written as a source of information only. The information contained in this book should by no means be considered a substitute for the advice of a qualified medical professional, who should always be consulted before beginning any new diet, exercise, or other health program and before taking any dietary supplements or other medications.

The author and the publisher assume no responsibility for any adverse effects arising from the use or application of the information contained in this book.

Products, pictures, trademarks, and trademark names are used throughout this book to describe and inform the reader about various proprietary products that are owned by third parties. No endorsement of the information contained in this book is given by the owners of such products and trademarks, and no endorsement is implied by the inclusion of products, pictures, or trademarks in this book.

FIRST EDITION

Library of Congress Cataloging-in-Publication Data
is available upon request.

ISBN 978–0–06–211700–7

12 13 14 15 16   RRD(H)   10 9 8 7 6 5 4 3 2 1

To the inspirista within
every woman

Contents

BALANCE YOUR LIFE, BALANCE THE SCALE

Introduction

Welcome to the most unconventional weight loss book you'll ever read!

Wait—let's stop there. To be honest, I kind of cringe at the thought of this being a weight loss book, because I firmly believe that we are *so* much more than numbers and that what really matters in life is who we are, not what we weigh. But I understand that you probably picked this book up because you'd like to be healthier and weigh less. I get it! I am very grateful that you are here, and I am excited to share my story and what I've learned from working with thousands of women just like you.

So even though we're not calling this a weight loss book, it definitely *is* a book that will help you release weight. What's so unconventional about it is that it will tell you to stop dieting, to eat what you love, to ignore the numbers on the bathroom scale, and to change the way you think about controlling your weight. And, unlike most books about weight, we won't be spending tons of time talking about what to eat. Instead, you'll learn about balance, which will help you kick dieting and self-loathing to the curb.

Listen, I know what you're thinking: *Balance, schmalance.* You don't care about balance. You just want to get rid of some extra pounds and fit into the jeans you wore five years ago.

I understand that you want to start getting results instantly. I know how that feels. I am a recovered yo-yo dieter, and I purchased so many diet books, I could probably open a bookstore with them all.

I used to joke that I could teach weight loss classes because I knew so much about nutrition and diets from reading so many books and doing so many diets. Many of the women I meet say the same thing—they're pretty sure they know what to eat, but for whatever reason, they are not committing to their health. And what's more, I find that the reason has much to do with the way we live.

Let me explain, I've worked with many women—and I realized pretty quickly, most of us have an idea of how to be healthy, right? I mean, we know that a blueberry is a healthier choice than a potato chip, and if weight was really the only issue, why would we even want to eat a potato chip instead of a blueberry? So, it's not really about the food (maybe a little if you are skewed by having done too many diets—we'll get into that later). And I also realized that women (and here's a lightbulb) do too much. We are living in a world where we are taught that "more" is better when it comes to schedules and stuff, and "less" is better when it comes to our bodies . . . and it can feel impossible to simplify when life has become increasingly complex.

I'm not talking about "balance" in the sense of perfectly juggling all of the balls in the air—striving for that type of balance has only made women more stressed, gain more weight, and feel like more of a big, giant failure.

Years ago, I began asking the women I worked with a very simple yet important question, "What do *you* want?" And this led to the development of my B.A.L.A.N.C.E. Program, which will assist you in redefining your own meaning and method for balance, based on something most diets simply cannot factor in—YOU.

So, by opening this book, you've taken your first step on the journey toward balancing your life and the scale. And you'll never go on a diet again. Congratulations, your dieting days are over!

Now, you're probably wondering why I am *so* anti-diet. Because diets (in and of themselves) simply don't work. Sure, if you lived in a bubble and were only focusing on following the diet with access only to the foods of the given diet—of course, that would work to help you lose weight, but think about these two very important factors:

1. You don't live in a bubble, and even if you did for a period of time, eventually you'd have to join in "real life" again. It's impossible for a "bubble" to factor in your life realistically.

2. Would the weight loss alone really make you happy and fulfilled?

If you want to live a healthy, vibrant life, you've got to move away from the crazy "on-and-off" world of diets and embrace balance and self-love instead. My life's mission is to help all women (including myself) rediscover who we were each born to be, find balance, embrace our uniqueness, connect with each other, overcome fear, use our gifts, feel weightless, and smile a lot along the way. Helping people do all this is one of the goals of my life and of this book.

Balance Benefits

Believe me when I tell you that when you choose to live your life by being in balance, you will release weight—both in your life and on the scale. No gimmicks. No starvation. No impossible exercise plans—just a balanced approach that will improve every single part of your life. Being in balance reduces stress, and reducing stress helps you lose weight. It's that simple. I know this because I've seen it happen for thousands of women, starting with myself.

Thirteen years ago, I overcame borderline diabetes and lost more than a hundred pounds, ironically when I decided to ditch dieting and all of the self-loathing that goes with it. Sure, I exercised and chose nutritious foods. But there was way more to it than that—that was just the beginning. I lost all that weight (and have kept the scale in balance for over a decade) by making a far more fundamental change than just cutting down on calories—I transformed my life by learning what it meant to actually love myself. I changed myself from the inside out—I found my anchor to keep me in balance. And by being in balance, the scale balanced itself. You will learn all the intricate up-and-down details of my story throughout this book, as my story is intimately connected to my B.A.L.A.N.C.E. Program.

Over the past decade, I have devoted my life to assisting other women in doing the same thing. As a certified wellness coach, author, blogger, consultant, speaker, workshop teacher, and Curves fanatic, I have helped women release weight and find happiness by learning how to restore balance to their lives.

Take Donna, for example. When I met Donna, she was exhausted, drained, and stressed out. She'd been trying to lose her baby weight for twelve years and had been on every diet imaginable. Her calendar was booked day to night with housework, a part-time job, carpooling, soccer games, and ballet practice. Her husband was working and traveling all the time, yet they were barely able to make ends meet. She rarely saw her friends. Although she used to pride herself on the way she looked, she hadn't worked out in years. She felt out of shape, out of touch, and completely out of balance.

Sound familiar?

With my guidance, Donna redefined her own meaning and method for a balanced life that in turn balanced the scale. She lowered her stress levels, increased her commitment to taking care of herself, and reconnected with friends. And guess what happened after all that came together? You've got it—she lost the weight she'd been unhappily carrying around for more than ten years. Like so many of the women I've worked with, Donna learned that the more you're in balance, the less stressed you are, and the less stressed you are, the easier it is to release weight.

Many of the women who come to me for help are unhappy with the way they look and feel. They beat themselves up for just about everything. They are juggling a million responsibilities, but they still feel empty. They come from all different backgrounds and every age group, but they all tell the same story: They want to feel better about themselves, but they are blocked by exhaustion, frustration, self-anger, and disappointment. And they feel totally out of balance.

I have spent the past ten years developing and fine-tuning my B.A.L.A.N.C.E. Program and in the process have assisted thousands of women in achieving inspired weight loss (and keeping the weight off) as a benefit of restoring balance to their lives. The program even offers balance techniques for when life inevitably throws some curveballs.

The B.A.L.A.N.C.E. Program has grown in leaps and bounds over the last decade. It didn't just happen overnight—and quite frankly, neither did my personal transformation. The techniques and program have evolved through the influence of my own life experiences as well as those of the women I've worked with. I've learned from every one of them. For all of us, this program succeeded where *so* many diets had failed. Now I'm thrilled to be taking the next step and putting my B.A.L.A.N.C.E. Program into a book that will reach more women than I could ever connect with in person.

Although my B.A.L.A.N.C.E. Program does indeed help with weight loss, it's so much more than just a weight loss plan. Most of the women I meet say they want to lose weight. But once we start talking, we find balance issues or sturdy roadblocks that prevent them from being the magnificent women they were born to be. So instead of putting on diet blinders and focusing on cutting things out, we look at the larger picture of their lives—their careers, their relationships, their priorities, and their dreams. Once they start utilizing the balance techniques to find balance in the other parts of their lives, weight loss happens organically.

It works the other way too. Recently a woman sought me out because she was having trouble with her business. Using the balance techniques, we solved her business problems—and along the way she lost fifteen pounds. She wasn't even trying to lose weight!

I'll tell you many more stories like these in the chapters that follow. Over the years, the women I've met have taught me so much, and I know you will enjoy hearing about their triumphs as well as their struggles.

Now that you know a little about me and how I formed my B.A.L.A.N.C.E. Program, it's time to begin defining your own meaning and method for a life in balance.

I'm so excited for you—you're about to begin one of the most exciting journeys of your life.

Let Your Journey Begin

The journey in between what you once were
and who you are now becoming is where
the dance of Life really takes place.

—Barbara De Angelis

The journey on which this book will guide you is about you: your life, your values, your body, your health, your mind-set, your happiness. It's about you being the most passionate and energetic version of yourself possible, using your unique gifts and talents to care for yourself and serve the world.

In the pages that follow, you'll discover everything you need to bring balance to your life. My highly successful, highly rewarding B.A.L.A.N.C.E. Program will provide the tools, vision, step-by-step guidance, and inspiration you need to find balance and lose weight.

Using the B.A.L.A.N.C.E. Program in this book, you'll learn how to:

- Explore and envision what would truly make you happy, and use that vision to define your own specific balance goals

- Define your own meaning and method to finding balance in life and with the scale—releasing dead weight off your shoulders *and* your body

- Use fun worksheets and quizzes to help you become an expert

- Start restoring balance immediately by finding humor in your unique imperfections and embracing them

- Discover the most effective ways to set and reach goals

- Practice self-care in realistic, practical ways

- Overcome obstacles by taking my no-excuses approach

- Use techniques to stay in balance no matter what changes, adversities, or curveballs come your way

- Use long-buried personal strength to fire up your energy, take action, and tackle change

- Unburden yourself of the negative assumptions that weigh you down and hold you back

- Make informed choices instead of sacrifices

- Most importantly, feel joyful instead of stressed

The B.A.L.A.N.C.E. Program

Being in balance is the key to releasing the excess weight in your life and your body. But balance is a state of being and a way of living, not an end point in and of itself. My B.A.L.A.N.C.E. Program is the result of many years of knowledge-gathering and working with thousands of clients. The program has seven steps, each with two focuses: a practical, long-term approach and a spiritual, everyday approach. In all there are fourteen techniques that you can use to redefine your own meaning and method for balance in life and on the scale.

The Practical B.A.L.A.N.C.E. Techniques can be used to create your own customized approach to finding balance. You can take a linear (step-by-step) path, or you can intertwine the techniques. You will learn all about them in more detail throughout the book, but in short, they are:

I've learned that balance (in the form of having all your ducks neatly in a row) is bunk, that we can each define our own meaning and method for balance, that we can set our own terms for success, and that real joy is not something that is dependent on circumstance or stuff.

✲ My No-Judgment Guarantee

I want to make something crystal clear right off the bat. In the past when I've read diet books, self-help books, and inspirational books, I've sometimes felt judged by the author. In most cases, that probably wasn't the author's intent, but with my self-esteem at an all-time low as I was reading, I pretty much thought *everyone* was judging me. Believe me, many women feel that way.

But I don't want this book to make you feel judged. That's why it comes with a **no-judgment** guarantee:

I do not think you need to lose weight. I do not think you are lazy. I do not think your life is a mess. I do not think you are ridiculous or emotional. I think you are perfect just as you are. You are beautiful inside and out. You are capable of more than you know, and you have everything you need within you to create exactly what you want for your life. You are a complete, whole, capable, resourceful woman.

I have been every size, from 4 to 44, and then some. I am far from perfect, and my intent with this book is not to make you think that I have the magic formula for you to lose weight. Nor is it to hypnotize you into believing that once you lose weight you will be more of a person. On the contrary, you already have all the answers you are looking for within *YOU*. I believe you have everything you need to be happy, healthy, vibrant, and alive in this moment, regardless of your shape, size, credit score, or list of past mistakes.

If your balance between life and the scale is making you less than happy, that's where I come in. I can help you find the balance you crave so you can live the life of your dreams. I am thrilled that you decided to take some time out of your life to read this book.

B Brain Dump and unclog your mind

A Assess and clearly understand your current state or situation

L Let Go of anything that does not serve you or the greater good

A Add In to enrich your life and help you create your vision

N Navigate the journey

C Confront issues along the way

E Engage in life and what you set out to do

The Everyday B.A.L.A.N.C.E. Techniques represent my balance mantra for life; they can be used every day to help bring balance to your life. When you are feeling stressed, chaotic, worried, hectic, frazzled, lost, or just not like your best self, try one of these seven techniques. We will go into more detail about why and how they benefit your life and help you release weight, but in summary, they are:

B Breathe

A Accept

L Laugh

A Appreciate

N Notice Nature

C Connect

E Experience

Figuring Out What to Eat

People who buy diet books usually jump right to the sample meal plan section—I know that's what I did when I was on the dieting roller coaster. This book is different. As strange as it may sound, although this book is about weight loss, it doesn't focus mainly on food.

I won't tell you what to eat, but I will help you create your own balanced approach to eating that will suit your life better than any off-the-shelf diet. But remember, the B.A.L.A.N.C.E. Program is all about *YOU*. If the structure of a fixed meal plan will help you along, go ahead and add it in. If the pressure of a diet weighs you down, go ahead and let go of it. I'll provide exercises that will help you determine what type of eating plan works best for you. Then we'll add in the techniques to personalize that plan and turn it into an effective tool for true lifestyle change.

Whatever you need to do to be the healthiest, happiest, most vibrant version of yourself possible is 1,000 percent okay with me, because I know in my heart that *you* have the power to change your life.

You Are an Inspirista

Inspirista. I came up with this term one day while speaking with a friend. She mentioned the word *fashionista*—a person devoted to fashion—and my immediate reply was, "I think I'd rather be an inspirista!" Then I sat down with my trusty notebook and pen and defined what that meant:

> An inspirista is a woman who has a positive attitude, an inner glow, and a contagious energy that makes others want to smile. She takes challenges in stride and doesn't allow a failure to hold her back or a risk to scare her off. An inspirista turns failure into success; her test becomes her testimony.

An inspirista finds and embraces beauty in herself. She lives every day to the fullest. She inspires people to live with love, to follow their passions, and she serves the world by using her unique gifts to help others.

Who Is the Expert?

As you begin your journey, please keep this in mind: I want you to think of me as your guide, not as the expert who will give you all the answers you need to solve everything that's going wrong in your life. It would be disingenuous for me or anyone else to ever make that claim. We are all unique individuals with completely different thought processes and circumstances. There is no one-size-fits-all plan for finding balance.

The word *expert* implies that person can swoop in, fix you, and make everything better. But I don't believe that you need fixing. It's fine to make changes and improvements in the choices you make and the way you think about life. Change is the essence of life. But you are not broken. You are exactly where you should be in your life journey.

I do, however, believe that I have guidance to share. I am a lifelong learner. I am constantly taking courses or reading, and I like to simplify things to make them easy to understand. From my years of experience working with thousands of women as well as all my training and self-study, I've collected lots of incredible advice. I can't wait to pass it along to you, because certain nuggets of gold need to be shared!

B.A.L.A.N.C.E. Rule #1: There are no rules. You set the terms. You define your success. You find your balance. You are the expert of you.

You have all the answers you need within yourself. You already have everything to live the life you want to live. I am happy to guide you through the process of finding balance, but I want you to realize that *you* are your own best expert. You have your own inner guide who is very powerful. You can and will create whatever you want for you—and I'll be with you every step of the way.

Chapter One

We Eat How We Live

The Food-Life Connection

We are indeed much more than what we eat,
but what we eat can nevertheless help us to
be much more than what we are.

—Adelle Davis

W hen my mother, sister-in-law, and I opened our Curves franchises in New Jersey in 2001, we had no idea what to expect. My mother was a hairdresser turned realtor turned Curves owner who had never before had her own business. I had worked for a pharmaceutical company, and my sister-in-law was an interior designer. Our skill sets were mixed, but we had one thing in common: our love for helping women.

My mother is a nurturer. She listens, empathizes, and drops everything to help anyone. When she was a realtor, she often would try to talk people *out* of buying homes because of the water in the basement or the noisy neighborhood or the crack in the foundation (and then she'd feel terrible if they went ahead and bought the place anyway).

She looked at every client as a member of her own family. Because of this, she had to leave the business. She had also developed tendonitis in her legs that was so bad she could barely walk a few feet without pain overtaking her.

My sister-in-law is a helper, a confidant, an advice giver, a problem solver—and as icing on the cake, she has a keen Stacy London–like sense of style. Danielle is my go-to wardrobe consultant.

Once I found out that my health was at risk with borderline diabetes, I got the huge wake-up call and forced myself to go to the gym (kicking and screaming) and to eat healthier foods. The diagnosis also made me realize something else—how little I was practicing self-love. Sure, I preached it. I was "girl power" all the way in college. I believed we should love ourselves no matter what (and I still believe that). But when I found out I was having blood sugar issues, I went to a nasty place of negative self-talk. I would never say the things I said to myself to anybody else. At the time, Danielle and my brother were dating, and Rich was my antithesis when it came to working out. He owned a fitness center and actually won the title of Mr. World Fitness. He has certifications in personal training, nutrition, massage therapy, and exercise physiology. But then that lightbulb moment led me to seek my brother's guidance and begin nurturing myself in a healthy, balanced way. Rich taught me everything he knew about nutrition and fitness.

Rich and I are very close, but we were very different. I was born during a blizzard in 1976—I came out without so much as a doctor, an epidural, or even a fifth contraction. My mother was waiting for the doctor in the room, but I couldn't wait to come into the world. Just a few years earlier, my mother had been in labor with my brother for almost two days! He has always been the laid-back one, and I have been a bit more animated—either falling down steps and breaking my tailbone, running into the glass window at the store while rushing to buy presents, ripping my dress at my cousin's wedding, or being left at the prom. Yes, I was quirky, klutzy, emotional, and much more frazzled than my older, calmer brother. Sure, I laughed a lot, but he had an aura of Zen around him, while I always had a cloud of dust around me. Finding balance did not come naturally to me, or so I thought.

I took Rich's advice on fitness and nutrition, listened to my own inherent wisdom of practicing self-love, swore to my mother that I would never again ask her if my butt looked big, and set out on a quest to live life in balance. Releasing weight happened almost naturally—an added bonus when I dropped it as a goal and instead made a personal commitment to living well.

It was kind of ironic, and a bit shocking. I had always searched for some kind of magic pill to take off weight. But I learned there was no magic. I needed to eat healthy foods in moderate amounts and move my body regularly. There are diets that promise rapid results, but the test is in turning the diet into a way of life. And, really, if rapid results mean feeling deprived, exhausted, or focused solely on a number, what good are they? I'd still be unhappy whether I was a size 4 or 44.

If the diet approach you are trying doesn't make sense for you in the long term, if it's not a good fit for who you are or doesn't make you a happy, joyful version of yourself, then you've got to make a change. It isn't worth losing weight if you also lose the joy of living.

The magic is in the commitment, not a pill. The commitment already lies within you. Commit to being the woman you were born to be. Commit to the little girl inside you. Commit to vitality, not just weight loss. When you do, you will see a change in your body, health, and spirit.

I felt like I had the beginnings of a secret, an inkling that there was something more for us women to focus on than the scale and the size of our jeans. It seemed like God had opened my ears to hear my calling, because I couldn't go anywhere—a nail salon, a restaurant, a doctor's office—without hearing women agonize over their weight or their stressed-out lives. I felt like I had a secret that I just had to share: we don't need to spend all this time worrying; we can enjoy life instead and live well. Although I was still learning exactly what that meant and how to do it, I wanted to share this message with women and reinforce it for myself.

I also loved helping women (and still do). I think I was especially drawn to this at that time because we all tend to teach what we most need to learn, I needed to learn self-esteem. I'm a girl's girl at heart, and I have always wanted women to live to their full potential, which has led me to write about the meaning of life since I can remember. When I graduated college, I had the Eleanor Roosevelt quote, "The future belongs to those who believe in the beauty of their dreams," printed on my invitations and written in red icing on my cake. (Later, I even had that same quote painted on my daughter's nursery wall.) Even though, at the time, I still had some issues with my own self-esteem, I've always wanted women to feel good about themselves. So when my coworker Julie told me that she and her mom owned a Curves franchise, I realized I had found an opportunity to help women live a healthy, happy life and follow their dreams.

I was intrigued about buying franchises for many reasons. First, I had spent most of my life on some sort of diet. I was finally able to control my weight, but for years I had been on the dieting roller coaster. My highest weight was over 265 pounds, and I had released a hundred pounds since that time. Second, I hated working out, and although the thought of a thirty-minute full-body strength training and cardiovascular workout seemed impossible, it definitely was right up my anti-gym alley. Third, I thought it could help my mom with her tendonitis and perhaps be a business for us all, just as it was for Julie's family.

So the three of us ventured out to Julie's family's Curves, which was actually quite a distance from our homes. We joined, and we were hooked right away—and my mother's tendonitis started improving. Before going to Curves, she struggled to do simple things like food shopping or going to the mall. Soon after, though, she felt like her old self. She was moving again—she went from barely walking to being able to jog, jump, and even dance. This was the first workout my mom not only *could* do, but also *wanted* to do. With the upbeat music and friendly environment, my mom found a gym where she felt comfortable. Danielle and I felt the same way.

Before we knew it, we were on a plane to Waco, Texas, to learn all about business ownership from Gary Heavin, the founder of Curves. With my father and brother cheering us on and helping us get our facilities ready, this venture became a true family business.

Within a year, we were opening franchises of our own. Little did we know how much our lives would change, and that we were on the path to helping thousands of women transform their lives as well.

I became so passionate about my work that it became my mission. I studied and read books about health and wellness instead of dieting and weight loss because I wanted to understand everything I could in order to help myself and our members be the best, happiest, healthiest version of ourselves possible. Wanting to delve deeper into life issues, I took coaching courses at New York University and Spencer Institute. This launched a quest for balance, and I eventually became a certified wellness coach with a private coaching practice. Then I expanded my Curves classes into the community and started speaking at offices and corporations. I started writing again, contributing to newspapers, magazines, and websites.

I studied and practiced balance and spirituality, and then when life threw my family some major curveballs, I was able to put my studies to the test and even learn so much more through life experience. Today I'm married to my best friend, and I enjoy every fun-filled teary-eyed moment of being a mother to my precious gifts from God: Millana Elle (aka LuLu) and Ewing James (aka Little Man). I will share this all with you throughout the book, but let's begin with how I discovered the importance of food, far beyond its effect solely on the scale.

Looking Back

Because I have been every size from 4 to 44, I have spent much of my life labeling myself chubby, chunky, thick, heavy, and—my personal favorite—big boned. When I was in high school, I was somewhat able to control my weight by constantly being on a diet. In college, with a new schedule, new surroundings, new friends, and being away from

Inspirista Approved

Curves: Why It's Different, and Why I Love It

I'm not exaggerating when I say Curves changed my life. I first worked out at Curves twelve years ago. Since then, it's been with me through many major life transitions, including career change, marriage, two children. When we take new directions in life, we often have a hard time taking our workout with us. But Curves fits so seamlessly into life that there's always room for it. Curves is a major reason that I've been able to maintain a healthy body, stay strong, and live in balance for all these years.

Curves is a one-stop shop when it comes to women's exercise and nutrition. The company, which has thousands of locations in ninety countries around the world, is committed to helping women be healthy and strong. The world's leader in women's fitness, Curves is continually investing in research to provide members with the latest technologies, fresh strategies, and unique programs for living a healthy, balanced life.

One Word: Community

Curves is all about community. From the first visit, you can see that the people there care about you and your goals. From the circular setup of the circuit to the various contests, activities, and happenings in each facility, Curves truly facilitates a supportive environment of positive, inspiring women.

Promotes Strength, Confidence, and Self-Esteem

Curves isn't a facility that promotes starvation or thinness as the gold standard. On the contrary, Curves promotes strength, inner power, confidence, and self-esteem so that we love our bodies and take care of them well. The Curves mind-set is clear in its mission, "Strengthening Women," and is reinforced in its magazine, *Diane;* and online communities.

No Skimping on Your Body

In most gyms, you can choose whether to do cardio, strength training, stretching, or all three, and you can opt just to train certain muscle groups in an effort to do what's called spot reducing. But our bodies need all three types of exercise—cardiovascular exercise, strength training, and stretching—for total health. And because spot reducing is a myth, there's no point in wasting time on it. Curves sets you up for success, so you can't skimp on your body. By design, you work every major muscle group, check your heart rate at least three times during your workout to make sure it's elevated, and end your workout with a wonderful stretch.

No Men, No Mirrors, No Makeup Required

Sorry, guys. Sometimes a gal likes to work out without having to doll up or be in a gym filled with men. While watching your form in the mirror is crucial in a traditional gym, it can be discouraging if you are self-conscious. At Curves, a circuit coach is available to teach, check your form, and motivate, so no mirror is necessary. Being in a girls-only environment is comfortable and allows you to have ladies' night any day of the week!

A Complete Solution to Living Well

At Curves, you get more than a workout. Curves offers complete exercise, nutrition, and weight loss solutions to millions of members. Members are supported by a personal coach, which gives you the support—with fitness, nutrition, coaching, and motivation—you won't find anywhere else. There's even a focused ninety-day program during which participants could lose as much as twenty pounds of body fat and twenty inches.

To find out more about Curves and find a location near you, check out the website, www.curves.com.

home, my emotions were all over the place, and without awareness or knowledge of how to handle them, I began eating more and more. Throw in the fact that I was now free to go to Denny's at two A.M., and unhealthy habits became a natural part of my new life.

As others gained the freshman fifteen, I gained the freshman fifty— and then sixty, seventy, and eighty pounds! I subconsciously tied my worth to my image, and when my weight hit an all-time high—and my self-image was marred by nasty comments from strangers and having my belly rubbed one too many times as I was mistaken for a pregnant woman—I became desperate to lose it. I thought that weighing more made me less of a person.

That's when the yo-yo diets began. I tried everything to manage my weight, but it all played out the same way: lose it quick and gain it back quicker. It was an ongoing joke with my friends and family: "What diet are you on now?" "Can you eat carbs this week?" My life and food choices were ruled by whatever diet du jour I was following.

After college, my emotions stabilized a bit, middle-of-the-night diner runs ended, and the yo-yo diets calmed down. But my lifestyle was centered around work, busyness, stress, and social activities. I lost some of the college weight but was still allowing my lifestyle to dictate my eating patterns, and my eating patterns to dictate my lifestyle. Instead of mindfully and consciously choosing healthy foods to stay energized and be healthy, I ate as an afterthought with little consideration for the amazing power that food has not only to fuel my body but also to energize my life. Although I knew what healthy food was, I didn't choose to eat healthfully because I didn't know how it would impact me other than on the scale.

Making the Connection

To be honest, I gave up caring about my weight because I had obsessed about it for so long, by that point it was easier not to focus on it. And so I didn't. Until one day, I got a huge wake-up call. I passed out while shopping at a local mall. When I came to, I ran to the cookie stand and gobbled up two chocolate chunk cookies and a carton of milk. I felt better but knew this was not normal. I worried that something was wrong. My fears came true when I found out I was having blood sugar issues. If I wasn't careful, the doctor said, I could easily wind up with type 2 diabetes.

Of course, I immediately went to the place of blame, beating myself up. What was wrong with me? How could I let this happen? When I stopped the negative self-talk and digested the news, I realized there was a disconnect with the way I practiced self-love. I was starting to see the effect of not nurturing myself well—the impact that food had on my life, beyond the number on the scale—and I didn't like how it felt. For the first time in my life, I began to recognize that food played a much more significant role than I was giving it credit for.

When I look back on that period, I see so clearly the distinct correlation between my eating patterns and my life. I now call this the food-life connection. It's basically the simple fact that we eat how we live.

Balancing and restoring my food-life connection was an integral part of changing my body inside and out, and overcoming the threat of diabetes. When our food-life connection is *in balance,* we eat food for its intended purpose. We eat what we need and enjoy without overeating or bingeing. There is a deep, soulful connection between food and life, and our weight lines up with where it should naturally be. The foods we eat energize us, improve our mood, and enhance our ability to focus, which helps us effectively communicate with and listen to others. We choose foods that protect our bodies from disease, shield us from the negative effects of stress, and can even reverse signs of aging both internally and externally.

When our food-life connection is *out of balance,* we eat foods for many reasons other than simply fueling and nurturing our bodies. We may be eating as an afterthought, just trying to get through a busy day and running to pick up whatever food we can find. We're working longer hours, our kids are in more activities, and we have packed schedules with little or no time for healthy behaviors. Or we may even turn to food almost like a drug in an effort to feel less anxious, sad, lonely, bored, and defeated. When our souls feel empty, we desperately try to fill them. Because we are constantly surrounded by food, and because eating gives us pleasure, we expect food to fill our emotional void; and when it doesn't, we keep taking in more and more food. Not surprisingly, body weight increases along with the weight on our shoulders and in our minds.

The food-life connection is circular: we must live well in order to eat well, and we must eat well to live well. But when our food-life connection becomes skewed, we lose balance in our eating habits, on the scale, and in our lives. I see this with women all the time when factors such as the pace of life, yo-yo dieting, lack of self-esteem, or simply not knowing what eating healthily truly means, create an imbalanced food-life connection.

Take Sara, for example. Sara squeezed eating into her jam-packed day. It was a necessary evil, an answer to a growling stomach, or a response to her frazzled schedule. Or she ate junk when she felt stressed, bored, angry, lonely, or depressed. She ate foods with little to no nutritional value, constantly felt exhausted, and couldn't lose weight—and she had not a clue why.

Tune In and Relax

Here's a great reason to find your balance: A 2011 study by researchers at the University of California, San Francisco, found that reducing stress—especially cutting back on stress-eating—was associated with reductions in abdominal fat in some subjects. The researchers believe the reason for this is that stress causes the body to release the hormone cortisol, and cortisol promotes the accumulation of belly fat, which raises the risk for type 2 diabetes and heart disease. I love the message this study sends: being in balance may help release some weight—and protect your body too.

Sara slowed her metabolism down with unhealthy eating patterns dictated by her overstuffed to-do list. She had no time to exercise or strength train, which contributed to her slow metabolism and made weight loss nearly impossible. And what's more, because her food had very little nutritional value, she felt sluggish and tired.

When Sara began learning how to balance her food-life connection, she immediately felt lighter. With good food, exercise, and a more balanced schedule, Sara's metabolism sped up, her fatigue notched down, and she finally started having the energy to consciously create the healthy, happy life she so desperately wanted. Nurtured in body and spirit, she lost weight naturally.

Your Food-Life Connection

Restoring balance to your food-life connection is not about depriving yourself through dieting. On the contrary, it's about recognizing the amazing power of food and the connection between food and life. It's also about using that knowledge to consciously make the best choices on your plate and in your life. When your food-life connection is healthy and balanced, you can enjoy your food and have fun eating without expecting it to fill your emotional emptiness. It's okay to love food! With its amazing natural powers, food can be healing *and* serve as comfort when you take time to lovingly prepare a dish for yourself or someone else. I am a total foodie—so much so that I married a chef. I say *love it* in context—as something that provides fuel, energy, delicious taste, and an enjoyable sensory experience that's often shared with family and friends.

By understanding the food-life connection, and by exploring and restoring your own personal food-life connection, you begin to use food in ways that are more physically and emotionally healthful. You can use food as fuel for your body *and* as fuel for your life in a balanced way that nourishes your body and your soul.

You can transform and rebalance your food-life connection by taking five very important steps, which I will explain in the following pages.

☼ Create a B.A.L.A.N.C.E. Journal

Throughout this book, I'll be asking you to do some written exercises, jot down your thoughts, and answer some questions. I recommend that you create a B.A.L.A.N.C.E. Journal for these activities and save the worksheets you create for use in later steps of the B.A.L.A.N.C.E. Program. Whether you use an inexpensive spiral notebook, a fancy leather-bound journal, or your laptop computer, writing is a crucial part of your balance journey because it gives power and perspective to your thoughts. It also allows you to gather and record feelings, observations, self-discoveries, and answers to questions in a place where you can easily go back and review, reflect upon, and explore them. You will learn a lot about yourself by looking back at the entries in your B.A.L.A.N.C.E. Journal.

Food–Life Reconnection Step 1: Ditch the Dieter's Mentality

The dieter's mentality is like a giant cinder block that knocks the food-life connection off-kilter. It forces us to put our lives on hold as we start diet after diet, and to believe that our happiness lies in a pair of size 4 jeans rather than within ourselves. Ditching that soul-sapping mentality frees you to look at food in a whole new way.

Instead of viewing food as fuel for life, dieters see food as the enemy. We use a designation system that labels some foods as good and others as bad. A good food implies that it helps you lose weight; a bad food implies that it causes weight gain. But food does *so* much more than control the number on the scale. Food is not the enemy. It is our fuel source, our friend, our energizer.

During my years of yo-yo dieting, my whole life revolved around my diet. My house was filled with all kinds of diet paraphernalia—books, machines, treadmills turned into coat racks, waist bands, sweat gear—you name it. If I thought it would help me lose weight, I bought it.

Whenever I started a new diet, I would begin with the best of intentions. I'd be struck with the thought that my weight was out of control and that I had to do *something*. The thought usually occurred on a Thursday and would immediately be followed by another thought: *I can't start a diet on Friday. It's the weekend and just an awful time to start! Monday is perfect. I will get myself ready, stock up on diet food, and launch my diet on Monday.*

In anticipation of the deprivation to come, I would fill up on Friday night, splurge all day Saturday, and on Sunday have the Last Supper—you know, the feast before the diet, the final French fries, the last luscious licks of ice cream.

On Monday, my weight would mysteriously be up five pounds from the week before, which would make me feel ashamed and guilty. Filled with zeal, I would follow my new diet to the letter and constantly feel famished. On Tuesday I would be so hungry I felt like I would faint from hunger, but I could make it through. But by Wednesday I'd be completely frustrated because the numbers on the scale had barely budged, and they certainly did not equate with the pain of the diet and the longing for a peanut butter cup or a slice of bread. So I'd start to cheat, fall off the diet, and feel terrible about myself. Before I knew it, I would start dieting again. It was a vicious cycle.

Week to week, month to month, year to maddening year—this is the Dieting Wheel of Frustration. The dieter's mentality overtook me, and food became my greatest adversary, my most cunning nemesis.

When you're on a diet, the dieter's mentality rules your life. You just don't breathe the same—when you start your diet, you seem to hold your breath until you cheat, and when you go off your diet, you let out all the air you held in since you started the diet. Of course, it's not the diet itself that causes this—it's our dieter's mentality. This mentality explains why the gym is usually much busier on Mondays than on Thursdays. It also explains why most women gain back the weight they lose on diets.

In the dieter's mentality, everything comes down to weight. You are either on or off, up or down, dieting or cheating. The dieter's mentality pushes eating food for health and vitality out of the mix. Tunnel vision limits you to eating for the number on the scale. This mentality clogs your brain and clouds you from being conscious of food's intended purpose. It's time to ditch the dieter's mentality in order to embrace your true food-life connection.

Letting go of it is a process, so let's begin with some simple words. I suggest you remove these from your vocabulary:

Start: as in, "I will start again on Monday." Remember, we don't need to **start** or **stop** or go **on** or **off** anything. We just need to live and live well. Live like the person you want to be. Begin now and never end. We all make healthy choices and unhealthy choices—that's part of life. If you choose something unhealthy, don't decide that you've ruined your eating for the day and will start over tomorrow, next Monday, next month, or next year. Focus on now! Flush away your regret with a few glasses of water and some movement and make the next choice healthier—which leads us to the second dieter's mentality word to ditch . . .

Bad: as in, "I was bad because I ate a cookie." We all do this. We eat, and we feel guilty. It's unnecessary! Following a bowl of ice cream with a huge serving of guilt does you no good. Not only does it take away the pleasure of the ice cream, but it prevents you from building balance into your diet and creating an eating strategy that leaves room for ice cream and other foods you love. Guilt drains you and gives you nothing in return.

Instead of feeling guilty when you eat something in excess, do something about it. Drink some water. Get moving. Did you eat a piece of cake? Dance around the room for a half hour. Have a few French fries? Do some squats in the shower or lunges up the stairs. Hot dogs at the ballpark giving you a tummy ache? Water with lemon all day long will make you feel much better.

In the following chapters, I'll help you learn to let go of the guilty feelings associated with self-care, food, exercise, and other choices that contribute to your well-being. Feel bad if you rob a bank, not if you eat a cookie!

Wait: as in, "I'll wait to buy new clothes." Or "I'll wait to go to the beach." So many of us believe that we can't start enjoying life until we fit in our skinny jeans. This presents itself with phrases such as: *I'll wait to go shopping until I lose five more pounds. I'll wait to start dating until I feel less embarrassed about the size of my butt. I'll skip this year's high school reunion and wait to go next year, when I'm back to my high school size.* Forget all that waiting. You are complete and perfect now. Stop putting your life on hold. Put a big smile on your face and start living. The single most attractive quality about any person I've ever met is the smile—the genuine, from-deep-within smile that you see when someone laughs out loud and is happy to be alive.

One Last Thing

The dieter's mentality is notorious for making us feel *less than* when our size goes up. Remember, your clothes size does not determine your value as a person. I know this isn't easy to accept, especially when you're constantly bombarded with media images of "perfect" women or when you hear about a celebrity who is considered fat because she now wears a size 6. Even though it's natural to sometimes feel imperfect, you must remember that you are a person of value no matter what you weigh. You are beautiful and unique exactly as you are. Your body is nothing to be ashamed of, and it definitely shouldn't stop you from enjoying life.

Once you ditch the dieter's mentality, change your vocabulary, and accept that you deserve to nourish your body and mind, you can just breathe and start to kick the yo-yo diets to the curb.

DRINK SOME WATER AND JAZZ IT UP
The Wonders of Water with Lemon

Drinking water is probably one of the best things you can do for your health. It has a huge, huge impact. One of the very first things I recommend as you set out to balance your life and your food intake is to drink water flavored with fresh lemon. This simple, positive action benefits your body in two ways.

First, if you are dehydrated—as many women are—drinking water with lemon helps you nurture your body by recognizing, respecting, and fulfilling one of its most basic needs. Every organ, tissue, and cell in your body needs water to survive and thrive. You will actually begin to feel more energized, vibrant, and alive as you rehydrate yourself.

Second, drinking water with lemon flushes toxins from your body by helping your kidneys, circulatory system, and sweat glands effectively get rid of unneeded chemicals, waste, and by-products. You will feel less bloated, experience less retention, and all-around feel a little lighter just by drinking H_2O.

Not only is it necessary to hydrate the body (which is roughly two-thirds water) and flush out toxins, it is vital to:

- Carry nutrients to our cells

- Absorb nutrients better

- Lubricate the joints

- Get rid of bloat (yes, if you need water you retain water)

- Keep body temperature regulated

- Rev up the metabolism

If you don't get enough water, it's not a matter of just being thirsty. It wreaks havoc on your body and leaves you feeling just plain lousy. If you want to live with energy and passion, you have to stay hydrated. Some of the side effects of dehydration include:

- Decrease in energy levels and fatigue
- Migraine (enough said)
- Major digestion issues, which leave toxins in the body
- Retained water that can lead to kidney problems

So go pour a glass and then keep on drinking! I know there are many prepackaged fancy water alternatives, but they're not necessary. Sixty-four to seventy-two ounces of clear water with fresh lemon every day will give you the maximum benefit.

Don't worry! You can jazz that plain water up yourself simply by adding some citrus (squeeze in some fresh lime, grapefruit, even orange) and mint. Or you can add drops of pure pomegranate or cranberry juice and a mint leaf. If you need a little sweetness, add a pinch of stevia.

How much water should you drink? That depends on how much of a water drinker you already are. If you usually never drink water, you can't suddenly start gulping down half a gallon a day. Gradually add it into your day. Choose water with lemon instead of soda, sugary juices, or iced tea. Keep a bottle of water with lemon in your workspace and your car, and drink frequently. If you're not drinking water at all, begin with at least thirty-two ounces a day and go up from there. If you're already drinking some, increase it to sixty-four to seventy-two ounces a day.

Food-Life Reconnection Step 2: Educate Yourself

It's kind of funny: even though I was a champion diet book reader, I actually knew very little about how food impacted my body. I knew how it affected the scale, and I would often label foods as good if they helped me lose weight or bad if they contributed to weight gain. The foods varied depending on my diet of the moment. At one point, if I even looked at bread, I felt bad. At another point, eating pasta was good. I was so turned around by what the word *healthy* actually meant that I believed a seventy-calorie chemical-filled snack was the healthiest option based on calories alone. I often would fill up on foods that were actually not healthy, but I thought they were because they were labeled low fat or sugar free or diet.

Like the old me, you've probably done so many diets that you don't even really know what being healthy means. I get it! I've been there. But when I decided to get off the Dieting Wheel of Frustration for good, I realized I had to educate myself on what it really means to be healthy. I cracked open books and spent hours online learning about balance, happiness, and health. I decided it was important to understand how the body actually functions, so I learned about digestion, metabolism, and nutrition and why it's so important to drink plenty of water. I took classes on wellness and nutrition and started studying food labels, astonished to discover what junk I had been putting into my body for so many years. My brother, Rich, who is one of the healthiest people I've ever met, committed to sharing his knowledge of nutrition, health, and fitness with me. And of course, Curves gave me a wealth of knowledge and training about how the body works.

Throughout this book, I will share and explain what you need to know to reconnect with food in a healthier way. I will give you some very basic information and some suggested reading so you too can empower yourself with knowledge. And remember, although perpetual dieting can confuse us on what is healthy to eat, inherently our bodies know. We just have to tune in and listen. For now, let's begin with some basics.

Food and Its Function in the Body

If you understand how your body uses various foods, it's easier to make smart decisions about what to eat.

We'll start with **protein.** Protein is necessary for building and repairing body tissues, muscles, hair, and nails and is often considered your body's primary building block. Protein helps maintain muscle and keeps your metabolism humming. Lack of protein can contribute to lack of energy, bone density, muscle elasticity, and collagen. At normal levels, collagen helps keep skin supple and young looking. You don't necessarily need a lot of protein, but you do need high-quality protein.

Fat is an excess energy storage system as well as an insulator and lubricator. When food is not available, your body can continue functioning by burning fat. There are healthy fats and unhealthy fats. The healthy fats lubricate your skin, hair, nails, and joints. These fats protect your muscles and bones, raise your high-density lipoprotein (HDL) and lower your low-density lipoprotein (LDL) to create healthy cholesterol levels. Eat healthy fats but only in moderation because they are also high in calories. Good sources include: nuts, salmon, halibut, sea bass, tuna, avocado, flax, olive oil, and canola oil.

Unhealthy fats clog your arteries and are bad for your heart. Fats to avoid are trans fats, partially hydrogenated fats, saturated fat (found in meats and full-fat dairy products), and deep-fried foods. Hydrogenated fats are often hidden in low-fat foods. One of the worst examples of this is low-fat peanut butter. Manufacturers remove healthy peanut oil and replace it with sugar, chemicals, and partially hydrogenated oils.

Carbohydrates provide energy and fiber. Excess carbohydrates that are not used to fuel your body are converted to fat. Fruits, vegetables, and grains are excellent sources of carbohydrates. Fruits provide natural sugar, which is used for energy, and a variety of vitamins and nutrients that nourish your body. The fiber in fruits helps stabilize your blood sugar levels and promote healthy digestion. Fruits also have **antioxidants** that fight disease.

Grains provide fiber to cleanse the body. They also provide a long-lasting source of energy, or fuel. Whole, natural grains are better than processed grains. When a grain is refined or processed, it loses fiber and nutrients. Robbed of nutritional value, processed grains provide empty calories that raise blood sugar and turn to fat if not immediately burned. Whole grains are rich in fiber, which helps cleanse your body of toxins. Good sources of grains include: slow-cook (not instant) oatmeal, whole-grain cereals, couscous, semolina, whole-grain dense breads, brown rice, Wasa crackers, and wheat germ. Instant rice, oatmeal, and other grains cook faster, but that's because they are processed.

Weighty Matters

It's important to know that weight is not always an indicator of health. You may interpret some people as thin, but that does not necessarily mean they are healthy. And you may interpret some people as heavy, but that does not necessarily mean they are unhealthy. There is a difference between body weight and unhealthy, dead weight. Dead weight holds us back and weighs us down. So release the dead weight from your life and your body, and you will feel weightless! Bottom line: you can be healthy at any size.

Because grains are an energy source, remember that the **amount** of energy you need and **when** you need it is important. We generally don't need a bowl of oats before we go to sleep because sleep doesn't require energy, right? When we start the day in the morning, it's a different story. Here's a simple rule: unutilized carbohydrates are converted to stored energy, which is essentially excess fat on the body.

Vegetables provide fiber, antioxidants, and hydration to the body. They are filled with antioxidants and nutrients for your cells. Low in calories and sugar, they are "free" foods that you can fill up on. It's hard to overdose on veggies, especially the green, leafy kind. It's good to eat them raw, but they're great cooked too. After you begin eating them, your body will crave them more and more. Trust me.

I used to hate vegetables (chomping on celery and carrots alone didn't appeal to me at all). But as I began to learn about vegetables' life-changing, energy-boosting, balance benefits, I sought out new and fun ways to prepare them. I even shredded cauliflower (it had the look and texture of rice) based on a recipe someone shared. It changed my perception of veggies, and before I knew it, I was addicted! Now, my body craves veggies—they are my go-to snack of choice! Once you learn all of the benefits of eating vegetables presented in this book, I'm sure you'll learn to love them too.

If It's Not Fresh, It's Fast

I was surfing XM Radio and happened to tune in to Cosmo Radio right when two of my favorite hosts, Kenny and Taylor, were talking about their coworker giving up fast food for Lent. She didn't know if Pizza Hut would be considered fast food, and a hilarious debate began.

After a little research, Kenny discovered that Pizza Hut actually considers itself fast food, but he was on the fence about calling it that. As I listened to the debate, I started to think about what qualifies a food to be fast. Here's my thought: if it's not *fresh* food, it's *fast* food.

Even if a restaurant takes an hour to bring the food, if it's freeze-dried or prepared in a microwave or deep fryer versus on a grill or stovetop, it's fast food. Actually, many chain restaurants use food that's frozen and already prepped. Some even reheat foods with premade grill marks!

If you think about it, it just makes sense—how could a restaurant that has over a hundred menu items possibly make everything fresh? So when you're picking a place to have dinner, remember that less is more. Fewer items on the menu is generally a good indicator that the food is fresh.

Why is fresh food a better choice?

Well, number one, our bodies are designed to best digest food that is indigenous to the land around us, in its most natural state. Better digestion means better health. My really simple rule is: when we eat real food, we feel real good.

A balanced diet consisting mostly of fresh foods contains important nutrients linked to preventing moodiness, so we're less cranky. And we communicate better with each other when we're not in a food fog. We are focused, productive, and generally functioning as our best selves when we are fueled up right. Note: Eating fresh food does not mean eating like a bird. Extreme dieting—meaning too-small portions—often has the opposite effect, making us total crank pots.

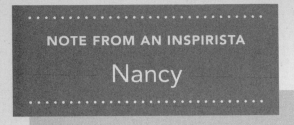

Nancy joined my 30-Day Challenge in July 2011. At the time, she had a full-time job and was juggling three to four part-time jobs along with being a go-to person for volunteer activities, all the while finding it difficult to be in balance. Here's what she says:

Since I began working with Jenn on the 30-Day Challenge, I have realized that diet and exercise alone do not work for me. What she has taught me is that I need balance in every aspect of my life—from cleaning out my closets and drawers to finding my inner happy child, journaling, and just taking the time to breathe. I have not only lost weight (9.5 pounds to be exact!), but I have also gained so much more perspective. I have eliminated aspects of my life that were weighing me down and have started to devote more time to me. As a busy person with multiple jobs, this was not an easy task. I reconnected with my love of cycling and cooking and even enrolled in culinary classes at the local community college. My weight loss results speak for themselves, but what you will also notice is what I gained: confidence, emotional strength, energy, and happiness. Thank you, Jenn!

Nancy

These are some of the most basic facts about healthy food; I'll share more as we go along.

Food-Life Reconnection Step 3:
Slow Down

As I mentioned earlier, I came into this world like a lightning bolt, and I spent the better part of my younger years in a rush for no reason—I was a bit of a stressaholic. My mother pointed this out to me a few years ago. "Jennie, honey, you can't sit still. You are always busy with something." I realized she had a point, but I was not alone. Most of the women I knew were the same way:

Busy. Strung out. Searching. Dieting.

Even when I could help our Curves members find more time to exercise, something else would cause their speed of life to increase. This speed would definitely affect the way they nurtured themselves, and it often dictated their food choices. If they got a job promotion, the celebration lasted only a minute, because soon they would be e-mailing at all hours of the night, wishing they had a lighter workload, waking up late, and grabbing a to-go bagel from a convenience store. If their kids were the star athletes, pride would soon be wiped away by exhaustion from the three-day Little League World Series, not to mention the parties, trophies, and drive-through dinners on the way home from volunteering in the clubhouse.

I realized the answer to really helping people—which I longed to do and was why I got into business in the first place—was encapsulated in what my mother said to me: help them stop searching and find balance.

The first lesson I learned on my quest was to **slow down.** The frenzied pace of everyday life plays a huge part in distorting your food-life connection. Thanks to nonstop advances in technology, we can print photographs in an instant, send messages with the click of a button, and cash a check without even leaving our computer. The call for convenience has literally taken over our lives and the way we look at food.

The downside to this crazy-busy lifestyle is that it leaves us tired and stressed. We're overextended and overworked, juggling a million things as we run from one responsibility to the next. And when physical or emotional hunger strikes, we're likely to appease it with a quick trip to the convenience store, vending machine, or fast-food restaurant.

The key to slowing down in a drive-through world is to first define your own meaning and method for balance in your life. Balance doesn't mean juggling dozens of balls and being terrified of dropping them. Choosing to be in balance means just that—making choices regarding which "balls" we actually want to hold on to, and which ones we choose to put down. You can begin by answering this question, "What do *you* want?"

Zen Quickie

A Minute of Meditation Goes a Long Way

Research shows that people who practice meditation and other relaxation exercises experience many health benefits, including reductions in blood pressure, heart rate, muscle tension, and levels of cortisol and other stress hormones in the blood. You don't have to meditate for hours to benefit from it. Even a meditative minute here or there can help clear your mind. Close your eyes in the shower, in the office, or whenever you're feeling stressed and take a few deep breaths. Inhale slowly to the count of four, hold your breath for the count of four, and exhale to the count of four. This quick and simple relaxation is just enough to both calm you and energize you.

I know, it's a tough question. But by answering it, you will begin setting your own priorities, listening to your heart over the chatter of your mind, learning to say no, and practicing self-care (don't worry—you will learn all about how to do these things throughout this book). By creating standards for your own behavior and the behaviors you tolerate from others, you clear junk out of your life. You begin focusing on the things that give you joy and dropping the things that don't. And, in doing this, you create time and space for healthy habits.

> We should all do what, in the long run, gives us joy, even
> if it is only picking grapes or sorting the laundry.
>
> —E. B. White

You can also slow down on a daily basis, taking a few moments here and there to mindfully focus on what you're doing—even when it's just a routine action such as drinking coffee or greeting a neighbor.

TAKE ACTION

PUT ON THE BRAKES

Choose to consciously slow down with everything you do: chew your food, savor your morning coffee, enjoy the steam of the shower, make eye contact and connect with every person you see (from the bank teller to your neighbor to your coworkers to your family members). Plan a home-cooked meal and get the whole family involved in preparing it. Take at least one regular responsibility off of your plate and delegate it to someone else. Create tech-free times in which your phone is shut off and your computer is out of sight.

Food-Life Reconnection Step 4:
Be Present

The next lesson I learned was the power of being present. You know how you feel when you are sick with a head cold? Tired, run down, dull, and not very productive. The same is true when you have a crowded mind filled with too much mental clutter. You feel tired, run down, and not very productive, not to mention harried, stressed, and inconsistent. These feelings have a negative impact on your food-life connection because they interfere with your ability to have a healthy attitude toward food and to make self-nurturing eating choices.

When your mind is crowded, it's stuffed with thoughts and worries about to-do lists, money, time, family, friends, the past, the future, and a million other things. The one thing that you're *not* thinking about is the present moment.

When you focus on now, rather than the past, the future, and all the things you've got to get done, you open up space to be clear, passionate, inspirational, and nurturing. It wasn't until I started practicing presence that I was able to truly listen to my own heart. There is infinite power in the present moment, but if you are too crowded mentally to appreciate that, you lose out on all that power. You miss beauty. You miss life. You miss opportunity. You miss connecting. You can eat an entire meal and not taste a single bite.

Being fully present in the moment is one of the best and most balancing things you can do for yourself.

TAKE ACTION

STOP AND FOCUS

To practice being mindful of the present, begin by focusing on what is immediately in front of you. Say it's a Starbucks coffee cup. Study it closely.

Look only at the cup—don't let yourself think about anything except the shape, texture, colors, and presence of the cup. Spend several moments blocking out everything else and noticing only the cup. Do this a few times to get the hang of it. Then, start trying it out on things that are a bit more important than a coffee cup—the sound of your child's laugh, the color of the sky on a gorgeous winter day, or the taste of a fabulous piece of chocolate melting on your tongue. Listen fully when speaking to others, pay attention. Be present while driving in the car, focusing on the drive and not on your mile-long to-do list. Keep practicing these mindfulness moments and eventually you'll start to feel more present without trying.

Become Aware When Your Mind Isn't There

Awareness is a first key to making a change. While practicing presence and being present can be overwhelming, I often suggest simply becoming aware when your mind isn't there with you in the moment. Then, use a visualization technique to bring you back to center. I have a couple of visualization techniques I like to use myself:

1. **The Three Lightbulbs:** Think of three lightbulbs. One is in a box in the cabinet, one is in the garbage recently burned out, and one is in the light fixture burning bright. The lightbulb in the cabinet has the promise of energy, the hope of light, but no actual power because it's not plugged in to a present-moment energy source. The lightbulb in the garbage has no power—its power is in the past, gone. The lightbulb in the fixture holds all the energy and power. When you become aware that you are not in the moment, visualize twisting in a lightbulb and watching a bright light appear when it's fully plugged in. That bright light is you, back to center, in this moment, where you have the power to create exactly what you want for your life.

2. **Driving in the Car:** Picture yourself driving a car. Imagine you are staring only in the rearview mirror. What will happen?

You'll crash into the car in front of you. Next, imagine focusing on three traffic lights ahead, way down the road. What will happen? You will miss the traffic light that you are approaching and possibly run a red light. Now, imagine driving a car and focusing on the road in front of you, using present-moment energy to push the gas pedal or pump on the break. Now you're in the present moment, rather than looking back at the past or forward into the future.

3. **A Snap Back in the Moment:** This visualization is very simple and is intended to pop you back into the moment. Snap your fingers. Hear the sound and remember it. Do it over and over so it is crisp, loud, and clear in your mind. When you become aware that you are not in the moment, snap yourself back to center.

To continue being mindful, you'll have to begin to free up space in your mind. We'll discuss this in greater detail in Chapter 2, but for now, if your mind is racing with thoughts, worries, and concerns, use your B.A.L.A.N.C.E. Journal to clear some of the clutter from your mind. What's swirling around in your head? What are you thinking about? Worrying about? What's sitting on your to-do list? Write it all down in whatever way feels best—there is no wrong way to do this. You can journal in prose, jot down bullet points, cut out pictures and create a cluttered-mind collage, or create a spreadsheet. The idea is to get your concerns out of your head and onto paper, leaving the space you need in your mind to be creative and insightful and live a passionate, inspirational, healthy life.

Food-Life Reconnection Step 5: Practice Self-Love

One Friday night last October, I went to a friend's house for a home-cooking/housewares party. I was looking forward to having a night out with the girls and doing a little shopping for kitchen gadgets—we were desperately in need of a new spatula.

The table was set with delicious finger foods, cheesy taco delight, crudités, spinach artichoke dip, and much more to sample. There was even a fresh—made-right-in-front-of-our-eyes-fresh—flatbread pizza with avocado, onions, and tomatoes.

Of course, over munchies and a catalog filled with recipes, the talk switched over to dieting. There were at least ten women in the room, so you know inevitably one woman would bring up guilt over what she should or should not be eating. One mentioned Weight Watchers, another was on a fourteen-day diet, another was cutting out all carbs. The comments were kind of hard to listen to. I mean, this was a room filled with fabulous, smart, beautiful women, yet they were so very hard on themselves over food. It was sad.

I realize that this same conversation happens everywhere, which is why I'm bringing it up in this book. It's not exclusive to these particular women who were at this party—I could have heard the same conversation in a nail salon, at the supermarket, in a restaurant, or in an office break room. Many women, regardless of their shape, size, or age, are judgmental of themselves. As a matter of fact, a recent study suggests that three out of four women are unhappy with the way they look. Three out of four!

It's funny because saying to someone, "You're beautiful just as you are! Stop the insanity!" doesn't really work. You get the face that says, "Oh, you're just being kind." The feeling can't be changed by words. Even as I'm typing this, I realize that words simply are not enough.

I believe we nurture what we love, so how can we love ourselves if we are constantly feeling like we don't measure up? We also love what we nurture, but to me the dieter's mentality of guilt and deprivation feels more like a whipping, definitely not nurturing.

I get it. Ten years ago, I would have been jumping right in with the madness. I decided to put an end to it when I realized that feeling like I wasn't good enough just led me down paths of self-destructive behaviors—completely out of balance. I decided I had to choose self-love instead, and then I spent time defining what it actually means to love myself. More than words, I had to choose behaviors that exemplified love and nurturing, such as:

- Stopping self-criticisms (i.e., asking, "Does my butt look big in this?")

- Practicing self-care, such as movement, exercise, eating well, resting, and being in tune with my body

- Living with passion and energy by using my gifts, helping others, serving, and relying on faith as an anchor

NOTE FROM AN INSPIRISTA

Denise

Denise joined my B.A.L.A.N.C.E. Program simply to learn a little about the notion of balance, and she knew I had an anti-dieter's mentality, which intrigued her. She had tried many methods of losing weight, even gastric bypass. While several of these methods worked for a while, something would knock her off course, and because she had the typical dieter's mentality of all or nothing, not only would her weight fluctuate but also her level of self-worth. She once told me that after a weigh-in, as the scale was going down, she and the women around her were celebrating her weight of 218 pounds—they were giving her high fives and all! She continued to lose a few more pounds, but then as life happens, she went up a couple of pounds a few weeks later—back to 218. This time, the same number garnered quite a different reaction. She said to me, "Jennifer, that same 218-pound mark—that just weeks ago had made me and everyone around me feel so elated—made me feel ashamed and guilty. The women even reacted with a sad pat on

- Creating a space that represents who I am from the inside out: free from clutter, awash in colors I love, filled with visual reminders and inspirations, and decorated with meaningful items

- Practicing love, forgiveness, and understanding of others so I could open up to being gentle toward myself. Life really is a mirror.

Self-love is a daily, ongoing practice. We all have days when we just don't feel great. But if we don't work at it, we allow what the media says or what we hear from others to make us feel like we are *less than* all the time. Like any other muscle, you have to strengthen your self-love muscle by choosing behaviors that exemplify what you mean when you say the words. I don't believe there is a right or wrong defi-

the back—and assured me I'll get there. I wondered at that point, where was I going? I am the same woman."

Since working with me, Denise has had several aha moments, which I will share with you throughout the book. Here's a note I received from her about the power of living well vs. living for the scale:

Recently I had foot surgery. I was very discouraged because I wasn't able to move as much. Although I was tracking my food and was exercising, I had two weeks in a row with a weight gain. I decided just to continue with what I was doing, though, because the benefits of healthy eating are now worth more to me than results on the scale. And to my surprise today at weigh-in, I lost 7.2 pounds! Before, I would have quit after two weeks of trying and then gaining. But this time I knew I wasn't going to change my way of eating because I would be giving up more than a number. I am glad I think like this now! I wish I had the same patience for healing my foot as I did for a good result on the scale!

Denise

nition; we must each individually define it for ourselves. Once we do that, we are kinder to ourselves—and each other.

Lack of self-love can skew the food-life connection dramatically. Often we don't take care of ourselves because we simply don't love ourselves enough. This comes up not only with my friends and in the world, but also all the time in the classes I teach.

After a recent class, a woman named Pat approached me and said, "Jennifer, I understand what you are saying about self-love. But I can't love myself! I've spent years trying to figure out how to. I've done the affirmations, focused on my best qualities, read books about it, worked with various people on it, and tried losing weight to feel better about myself, but no matter what, I just can't manage to love myself."

When we don't love ourselves, we think nothing of beating ourselves up and taking on guilt and shame. We hurt our bodies with yo-yo diets and extreme exercise regimens because we think we deserve to be starved and deprived. When we love ourselves, we nurture our souls and nourish our bodies. We love exactly who we are in this moment, choose foods carefully, keep our bodies in motion, and surround ourselves with people who support us.

That can be more easily said than done, as Pat has found. It can be very hard to nurture yourself if you don't love yourself. I know, I've struggled with this issue too.

When we nurture ourselves, we begin to love ourselves more and more. I see this time and again. After just one short week of nurturing herself, a woman named Ana said to me, "Jennifer, for the first time in a very long time, I like myself! I am proud of how I've taken care of myself. I am energized every day."

Here are some other ways to learn to love yourself:

Reach for your full potential. As women, we are sometimes conditioned to limit ourselves. Not because we are lazy or incapable— we do incredible things all the time, from working and raising children to managing schedules and providing an ear or lending a hand. But it's easy to fall into a rut. If this is true for you, pick a goal and begin to push yourself to achieve it. Take action beyond a daily to-do list of mundane activities and add in something soul stirring and challenging that you can commit to doing.

When Margie signed up for a sixty-mile weekend walk for breast cancer awareness, she had no idea if she could even do it. She hadn't trained for many years, and she had terrible issues with her feet. She knew she had 180 days to prepare, but she felt completely overwhelmed because she could hardly find time to do all her everyday chores, let alone hit the pavement to begin a proper training program. A few weeks went by when Margie did nothing to prepare. Then she began visualizing herself on the walk. She saw the sweat pouring down her face, felt her heart beating strong, felt the throbbing in her feet, saw her leg muscles pumping with every stride, and imagined feeling so much fitter, younger, and healthier. The next day, she started training. Once she committed fully to it, she found time. Five months later she finished the walk and never felt more proud, fearless, confident, and nurtured. Along the way, she lost forty-three pounds—without dieting.

Let your voice be heard. It's easy to shrink into silence in the corner of a room. When you have unexpressed feelings inside of you, you begin to fall into unhealthy patterns as a means to deal with them. Women who lack self-love often feel that no one cares what they have to say, so they just stop talking and may begin eating instead as a means to feel like they are silencing their own voice. I have done this many times in the past.

Communication can be difficult, but it's necessary that your voice be heard. When Marcia came to me, she had recently received a rude (and undeserved) dressing-down from one of her coworkers. Marcia didn't want it to turn into a blow-up fight, so she apologized. Her side of the story went untold, and Marcia felt awful about herself. She kept replaying her colleague's words in her mind and began to believe them to be true. She used food as a means to cope with her low self-esteem.

When Marcia and I discussed communication as a path to self-love, she resisted. "I don't know how speaking more often will make me love myself more. I think it will do just the opposite." Eventually, however, she chose to start speaking up, to thoughtfully allow her voice to be heard when she felt strongly about something or when she had something to share. She gave it a try at one of her staff meetings.

Marcia called me immediately afterward, and I could feel her glow through the phone line. She felt proud of herself for speaking up. Because of this, she committed to taking better care of herself and no longer silencing her voice with food. She began to release the extra weight from her body, but more importantly, a whole new world emerged where she felt confident to openly say what had been trapped inside of her for so long.

Self-love and nurturing breed confidence, and once you're confident, you can do anything. Self-love sets a good foundation for you to take care of all the other people and responsibilities in your life. Self-love improves relationships, it helps you communicate better, and it allows you to set high standards for the behaviors you tolerate from yourself and others. A woman who loves and accepts herself—flaws and all—is fearless.

TAKE ACTION

SELF-NURTURE STRATEGIES

There are so many ways to nurture and fall back in love with yourself. Pick one of these suggestions, or choose one of your own, and start nurturing!

- Go for a walk with your best friend.

- Share your thoughtful and honest feelings about something.

- In your B.A.L.A.N.C.E. Journal, write a list of your ten best personality traits.

- Massage your temples.

- Pour a glass of wine and take a hot bath by candlelight.

- Push yourself out of your comfort zone.

- Treat yourself to a bowl of fresh raspberries—and forget about what they cost.

- Close your eyes and think about something nice you did for someone recently.

- Make an appointment with your primary care doctor for a full physical exam.

- Play your favorite CD as loud as you like.

- Drink a tall glass of water with lemon.

- Ask your kids to empty the dishwasher while you put your feet up and relax after dinner.

Moving from Myth to Reality

There are so many balance myths floating around. When we buy into them, we feel more stress and we eat more, hence skewing the food-life connection even further. We carry more weight in our bodies and our emotions, and we feel unhealthy, tired, and dissatisfied.

Once you define and debunk your own balance myths, you can make healthier choices that will move you closer to balance (in life and on the scale) and give you a feeling of power and joy.

Here are some of the most common balance myths:

Myth: I have to attain perfection in order to be balanced.

Reality: Balance is not about having the perfect life, and the more you strive for that, the less fulfilled you will feel. There will always be gaps, and that's okay. Move with the positive, identify what you'd like to create, visualize fun ways to fill the gaps, and have at it! And if you find yourself faced with an imperfection beyond your control, embrace it and learn from it.

Myth: My life would be better if only . . .

Reality: Sure, it's normal to think about the if-onlys in life. If only you had more money. . . . If only you could work less. . . . If only you could lose twenty pounds. . . . If only you had time to exercise more. . . . The list goes on and on. Are you weighed down by a bunch of if-only thoughts? I call this the If-Only Syndrome, and I've found that it's a huge energy drainer. Instead of dreaming about if-only scenarios, focus on the joy that surrounds you and what you *can* do to improve your quality of life—this will naturally make you feel more in balance. We all have challenges in our lives, so keep moving forward, and if you have no clue what to do, be still and listen. Stillness is an action.

Myth: The grass is greener for everyone else.

Reality: Everyone has problems, worries, tragedies, and disappointments—even the people who are balanced and happy, without a care in the world. They may simply have learned how to put difficulty in perspective and to find joy from within. If the grass looks greener, remember, it takes work to keep that grass green too. Look at the land beneath your feet and get to tending. Green-Grass Syndrome can skew your thinking, make you bitter, and throw you completely off balance.

Myth: It's selfish to care for myself.

Reality: Self-care is not selfish; it's necessary. Think about airlines—they always say if you have a child on board with you, in an emergency you *must* put on your oxygen mask first or else you won't be able to take care of the child. You take care of so many people— your family, partner, coworkers, bosses, neighbors. Human nature drives women to take care of others, but the most effective way to do that is to take care of ourselves too. It's a delicate balance, because if we take care of Number One too much, we become selfish; but if we ignore our own needs, we become exhausted, stressed, and re-sentful—and not a very good caretaker after all.

Myth: I have to have it all.

Reality: Being in balance requires you to accept that you must define what the term *having it all* means to you. You may have to let some things go if they are minute in the scheme of your life. Many women strive to succeed at everything. But true life success means defining the things that are most important to you, going after them in a bal-anced way, and releasing less important goals. You'll never be happy if you try to succeed at everything because it's impossible. Be clear with yourself about what success really means to you.

I also think success is a mind-set, and begins with recognizing we are successful every day with even the smallest of achievements. For example, some days I feel successful because I made a beautiful scrambled egg for LuLu or because I put the dishes away while they were still warm from the dishwasher. This is success for some of us, and we should recognize even the smallest of achievements. Accept-ing the small successes in our lives allows us to feel more balanced and joyful. If we feel like we can't do anything right, we continually spin our wheels but go nowhere.

Myth: I cannot, and should not, fail at anything.

Reality: I've had clients tell me they feel stuck in a rut and com-pletely out of balance, but fear keeps them at status quo. Truth-fully, most successful people aren't lucky; many have failed time and time again. But they've held strong to their vision and their faith, and they accept the inevitability of failure. Fear of failure can be debilitating because it blocks you from taking inspired risks. The setbacks, failures, mistakes, rejections—whatever you want to call them—are just amazing opportunities for growth, learning, or rerouting ourselves and our mission.

Myth: **Women are too emotional.**

Reality: No, we're not! I think men like to use this myth when they don't want to open up about something. It's true: men and women have different emotional responses. And generally women show emotions more readily than men. But always remember this: flowers need both sunshine and rain to grow. Happiness is great, but crying is normal and necessary sometimes, and stifling emotions is not healthy. Embrace your emotions and don't feel bad about having a good cry once in a while.

Summing Up

In this chapter, we've discussed the importance of reestablishing a healthy food-life connection. By doing this, you will see an improvement in energy, a new perspective on food as fuel for life, and weight loss on the scale. The activities I suggested included the following:

- Create a B.A.L.A.N.C.E. Journal.

- Drink at least thirty-two ounces of water with lemon daily.

- Reconnect with food for its intended purpose: to fuel and nourish your body.

- Become more aware of what you're eating: chew, taste, and savor your food with mindfulness.

- Build self-love by nurturing yourself.

In Chapter 2, I'll show you how to clear your mind of the junk that interferes with your life in balance and how to create a revived life vision.

Chapter Two

....

B is for *Brain Dump* and *Breathe*

The resting place of the mind is the heart.

—Elizabeth Gilbert

....

You're about to learn the first technique in the B.A.L.A.N.C.E. Program. It's time to begin redefining your meaning of a life in balance.

Before we begin, here's something to keep in mind. In the B.A.L.A.N.C.E. Program, techniques can be used in a linear (step-by-step) way, independent in and of themselves, or in any combination that works for you. For the purposes of this book, and to give a sense of structure to begin your journey, however, we will build from one technique to the next.

Brain Dump: Clear Your Mind and Examine Your Thoughts

I've been a journal keeper since kindergarten, a natural-born brain dumper. I grab a pen and paper whenever my mind feels heavy, and I use my words in ink to release the weight on my brain. I learn a lot about myself through my writing—it is a healing, cathartic process of self-discovery.

I think brain dumping is fairly intuitive: most of us know to at least write a to-do list when we have a lot going on. But I find that brain dumping solely for ourselves happens less and less as our responsibilities increase. Whether we've taken on an intense career or are raising a family or a combination of both, when we are busy, we simply don't prioritize brain dumping for ourselves.

Realizing I was on the verge of diabetes really hit me hard. I remember going through a beat-myself-up phase of putting myself down, wondering why I couldn't just get it together and take care of myself, and thinking something was wrong with me. But then I recalled a quote I received from one of my most thoughtful mentors: "It's your attitude, not your aptitude, that will determine your altitude."

Instantly, something clicked. I realized I was being mean to myself and that's why I wasn't rising above my health challenges, my food obstacles, my poor self-image, and my nasty self-talk. With this realization came a natural urge to brain dump, and so I did. I wrote my feelings, and at first it was cathartic. It was dismal, but it was a release nonetheless, and that felt liberating. I was learning about myself, so that was good too. Soon, though, I began to reframe my thoughts and to write in a more positive tone, using my mentor's quote about attitude as my guide and choosing to focus on that which I could control. It helped me turn my life around.

Being clear and present is so important for me—I function much better with an uncluttered mind. Even writing a to-do list is simpler and more meaningful when my mind isn't swirling. I once came across a list I wrote when I was distracted by a million thoughts and worries—one of the tasks was to pick up doof instead of food. How mixed up is that?

Over the years, I've seen the benefits that brain dumping has had for my clients as well. First releasing, then reframing, followed by some specific questioning. Brain dumping is an integral part to finding balance and being in balance, because the more you carry in your mind, the heavier you feel physically and emotionally. By dumping out the thoughts that weigh you down, you create time and space for the present moment. The more you release, the clearer you become. As we discussed in Chapter 1, being present helps you balance your food-life connection and use food for its intended purpose.

Brain dumping is a fantastic tool that allows you to pour out onto paper the worries, dreams, fears, hopes, regrets, and expectations that are swirling around in your brain. Once you've got them out of your head and onto paper, you can examine them and decide which ones to hold on to, which ones to reframe, and which ones to let go of. It can be a very freeing experience.

Also, brain dumping opens you up to believing in yourself. Somewhere tucked beneath layers of worn experiences, walls of limiting beliefs, years of juggling and balancing and nurturing others, somewhere inside is the real you, the woman you were born to be. She holds the memory of a victory, the lesson from an experience, the call of your purpose. You know that woman well. You just have to extract her memory from all that is clouding your view of her and bring her to the forefront. Remembering and recalling helps you bring her back to life.

Women are amazing. We handle so many things (brilliantly, I might add) on a regular basis. I've seen women overcome debilitating diseases, manage tangles of family finances, raise incredible children, turn passions into careers, and use their skills to help others—yet so many of us fail to recognize that we have the power within us to create whatever we want for our lives.

But that's about to change. You and I will work together to re-discover the woman you were born to be and fully recognize your unique talents, gifts, and strengths.

Brain dumping is a life tool, a technique you can use now and throughout your life to help you clear out all the junk that's clogging your brain in order to make space to live in the present moment, to believe in yourself, to finally hear what's in your heart, and to create a revived life vision. It's a little like taking all the furniture out of a room before you paint and redecorate. Doing a total brain dump will make you feel lighter than you've felt in a very long time.

Let the Brain Dumping Begin

When I meet with women for the first time, they usually ask where we begin. I tell them to start wherever they want and simply tell me what's on their mind.

After a few seconds of awkward silence, the floodgates open and the brain dumping begins. They pour out everything that's going on in their world, in no particular order, but always in a way that eventually connects stories, feelings, and diets from different periods of their lives like a crisscross puzzle.

I'd like you to do the same thing, and I've got a few tools that will help you get going.

First, we'll do a **free-form brain dump** just to get stuff out of your head and onto the page. Next, we'll do a **center your focus** exercise to shine a light on your strengths, abilities, and past successes to discover your strongest self. Finally, I'll help you **create your revived life vision.** Using a series of questions, you'll root out the true priorities and core needs in every circle of your life—physically, emotionally, socially, and spiritually.

Along the way, I'll ask you to write some of your thoughts and answers in your B.A.L.A.N.C.E. Journal, which will give power to your thoughts and help you draw important conclusions about yourself, your choices, and your life.

I'll also pass along some really helpful B.A.L.A.N.C.E. Tips that you can begin using immediately, and I'll introduce you to the first Everyday B.A.L.A.N.C.E. Technique: **breathe.**

At the end of this chapter, you'll have a much better understanding of who you are. Then in later chapters, we'll use some of the self-knowledge you've uncovered during your brain dump to develop a list of life goals, key motivators, and strategies to help you overcome the obstacles that stand between you, a happy life, and a healthy body from the inside out.

The Free-Form Brain Dump

The free-form brain dump is all about releasing. It's a process in which you pour out whatever is on your mind—your history with food, weight, self-esteem, and other challenges and obstacles you're facing in your life. The free-form brain dump process allows you to begin clearing your mind.

Doing a free-form brain dump is simple: grab your B.A.L.A.N.C.E. Journal and start writing. Include lots of details—dump everything out of your head and onto the page.

Where should you begin? Anywhere. Just start writing down what's on your mind. Write in any way that feels comfortable—lists, paragraphs, notes, a letter to yourself, diagrams, even drawings. Whatever works for you—there is no best way to do this—and there's no wrong way either.

There are only two rules in brain dumping:

1. Don't make judgments about yourself afterward.

2. Don't try to fix anything now. Free-form brain dumping is simply about releasing.

If a blank page scares you, here are some starter questions and thoughts to consider:

- What do you hope to learn from this book?
- How will a healthy self-image and/or body weight affect your life?
- What are your fears about change? What excites you about it?
- What are your thoughts about health, food, weight, and self-esteem?
- What do *you* want?

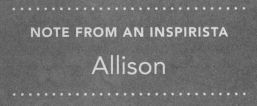

NOTE FROM AN INSPIRISTA
Allison

Jenn, I can't tell you what a difference writing has made for me. And I'm so glad you gave me the no-excuses approach. I avoided writing and brain dumping for many years because I was afraid someone would find it, and you know I have to keep everything private! When you gave me permission to write anonymously, I scoured the web looking for a tool that could help me journal in private, and I found an app for my phone that is password protected. Now I can journal anytime because it's right on my phone and I don't have to worry about anyone finding it! Thank you, Jenn, for opening me up to writing again. I feel much lighter, more like myself, and I am actually considering starting a completely anonymous blog with my journal musings!

Allison

As you write, allow yourself to be authentic and honest—no one else has to see what you're writing.

Don't even think about what you're writing, and don't worry about spelling, grammar, handwriting, or mentioning what you think you should feel rather than what you truly feel. Just release your feelings and let them flow.

Your goal right now is simply to get everything out and not to evaluate it or draw conclusions—yet. Don't be surprised if you make some pretty powerful discoveries right off the bat. If you experience an aha moment, let it happen. But more importantly, don't worry if it doesn't occur. Focus on freeing yourself to release the weight in your mind.

Here's an example of what one of my clients, Patti, wrote in her brain dump:

> *It is a difficult time in my life. I recently lost my dad, who I had taken care of for a long time. I can't fit into a lot of my clothes because I've gained weight over the past two very stressful years, and I don't have the money to buy new clothes. I lost weight years ago, but I gained it all back. I went through divorce, and when my mom died I became very depressed. Then when my dad got sick, I started feeling depressed again. I would say my worst time with my self-esteem was during my divorce. And through these difficult times—divorce, both my parents' illnesses—I was not eating healthy foods at all. I am now trying to focus on the positive side, and I am so glad I found Jennifer. Having female support is already helping me to stay healthy during a time of stress.*

When you are finished brain dumping, take a break. Go for a walk, make a cup of tea, have a meal, or even set your journal aside overnight. During your break, your subconscious mind will start processing what you wrote. You may even start to subconsciously reframe some of your thoughts. For example, one client who said she wanted to "get rid of the Pillsbury Doughboy rolls" on her back reframed the thought to wanting to have a strong, healthy back.

When you're ready, come back and read what you wrote. As you read, try to see connections, discoveries, common threads, and aha moments. What surprises you? What stands out? What troubles you? What elicits a deep emotional response? What observations and conclusions can you draw from what you wrote? Grab a highlighter and color anything that shows a facet of yourself that stands out. You may want to go over it several times or even read it out loud so you can listen to your thoughts in spoken form. If you want to explore anything more fully, go back and brain dump some more.

Many women who brain dump make some kind of self-discovery—and sometimes it can be surprising. When I met with Margie for the first time, she began brain dumping immediately. She talked about her job and how she often got mad at herself because she would get so

INSPIRISTA INSIGHT
Release Yourself from Fear

I know it's hard to just let go of fears, but by focusing on faith and hope instead of fear and despair, we open the door to all good things. Remember, where there is faith, fear cannot exist. Keep this in mind, and you'll be sure to untangle yourself from the worry web.

Being fearful is just another way we try to control our lives. It's like our hair—if it's curly, we work hard to make it straight, but one drop of humidity or rain makes it curly again. Life can be filled with so much more joy if we can cut our worry even just in half. So relinquish your fear and let go of all that negative energy. The happiness we feel when we are weightless is a catalyst for more happiness to be welcomed into our lives.

When we really want something, we tend to focus too hard on it. This means we get caught up in trying to figure out how to make it happen. We wait anxiously and anticipate results quickly, and if they caught up in the details that she would miss the big picture. She didn't even know what the big picture was most of the time, she confessed.

Soon she realized that she did the same thing in her personal life. If somebody did something to bother her, she would get stuck on that and forget the big picture or the real reason why they were having a conversation in the first place. All of a sudden, she said, "I think this happens with dieting. I get so caught up in the details of the diet, if I go off or something doesn't go as planned, I forget the big picture— that I actually want to be healthy and feel good about myself. Instead, I give up on the whole thing."

Margie realized that how she behaved in life and at work mirrored the way she behaved with food. When this realization clicked for her, she broke out into a huge smile. Little did she know, this discovery

---

don't happen, we get discouraged. If we work too much like a bull, we'll surely ram into stuff. All of this creates stress and negativity, and the response is echoed back to us with more stress and negativity.

Instead, detach from the *how*. Instead of working hard, work smart by taking inspired action. The operative word is not *if*, it's *when*. Be still and listen. The steps will unfold perfectly, as they should. Bumps become lessons, not blocks.

Take a little time to recognize the weight of your mind. What are you fearful of? Worrying about? Acknowledge it, and then do a visual exercise to wave good-bye to your fears and worries. Put them on a boat, sail them out to sea, watch them float away and disintegrate in your mind's eye.

Fear is static that prevents me from hearing myself.

—Samuel Butler

What Is Your Journal Personality?

If keeping a journal isn't working for you, maybe you're not using the right kind of journal for you. These categories can help you define your journal personality. Which are you?

THE JOURNALIST: You love to write and express your feelings.

Your best journal: A pretty notebook in which you can write everything—your daily food intake, your exercise and activity, your important occurrences, your feelings.

THE PROJECT MANAGER: You love tackling tasks and are considered a list master.

Your best journal: A three-ring binder. Use ready-made daily intake sheets or find templates on the web. Or design your own on your computer. Simply fill in your foods, beverages, moods, activities, and exercise in the template. Create to-do lists so you can tackle habits you'd like to create in your life.

THE COMPUTER GURU: Writing? You don't even own a pen! You love typing, and you are at the computer all day long.

Your best journal: An online journal you can plug in to, or even a spreadsheet file. You can even create graphs and pie charts of your daily intake and exercise.

THE ORATOR: You love speaking. You are on the phone all the time, and you have neither the time nor the interest in writing or typing.

Your best journal: A mini-tape recorder or video camera. Dictate your food choices, exercise, feelings, and other details. You can even take it one step further and create a video diary.

THE TECHIE: Writing, speaking, computers? Those things are antiquated! You use apps for everything.

Your best journal: An app that tracks everything on your phone.

put her on a transformational path, and just four weeks later, she had released years of weight off her shoulders and sixteen pounds off her body.

The other beautiful thing about brain dumping is it allows you to see your thoughts in black and white. Then you can choose to reframe your thinking, which allows you to begin to retrain your brain to look at things in a more positive way. Reframing opens you up so you begin to think (and choose) **possibilities** over **limitations, opportunities** over **challenges,** and you begin to focus on that which you can control as opposed to focusing on what you cannot.

Reframing was very important to Denise. When she brain dumped, many of her fears came out. She decided to take her fears and turn them into possibilities. For example, with her husband's pending layoff, she reframed it as a potential for her husband to take some time to relax, find a job that uses all his talents, and, overall, to stretch him out of his comfort zone. With this reframed perspective, Denise was beginning to feel excitement for the unknown as opposed to fear of it.

Brain Dumping as a Technique for Life

Brain dumping is a skill you can come back to throughout your balance journey and your life. You can use it whenever you're feeling stressed, overwhelmed, anxious, or out of balance. It's also a wonderful tool to use when you're facing an important decision or feel like you've hit some kind of a dead end in your life. The answers to so many of your problems and concerns lie within you. Brain dumping is a fabulous way to find those answers by clearing out the clutter in your mind and giving you time and peace to tune in to your innate wisdom and to listen to your heart. As you become more experienced with brain dumping, you may find yourself doing it naturally.

Writing is a very effective way to brain dump, but if being alone with a pen and paper scares you or isn't quite your cup of tea, finding a confidant to brain dump with can also be useful. Just be sure it's someone who can understand that brain dumping is just about clearing and releasing, not about debating or seeking judgment or advice.

If you're lucky enough to have an insightful, trustworthy confidant, ask her to help you by posing questions to assist you in self-discovery and reflecting back what you say. Hearing your thoughts spoken back to you is empowering and often leads to aha moments that clarify your thinking and inspire you to change.

If none of your friends or family seems right for this important task, consider scheduling a brain-dump session with a counselor, mentor, or coach.

Making Room for Now

We spend so little time living in the present moment. So often we are somewhere else—replaying something that happened moments ago, dwelling on past mistakes, worrying about the future, going over scenarios of what could/should/might be, or making comparisons with those around us. When all these not-now thoughts bubble in our minds, there is no room for now—the present moment.

Brain dumping is just one way to help you focus your energy on what's directly in front of you. Throughout this book we'll talk about other ways to peel away emotional clutter and live mindfully in the present moment. Learning to quiet the unconscious chatter in your mind allows you to listen better, think more clearly, experience life more fully, connect more effectively, make smarter choices, and enjoy the taste of food more. When you focus on the present moment, your senses are heightened and you feel more plugged in to life.

Foods That Help Clear Your Mind and Sharpen Your Memory

During the brain-dump process, it's helpful to eat foods that can help clear your mind and sharpen your memory. Yes, you read it right—certain foods can actually help with clarity and focus. For example, foods that are high in vitamin C, vitamin E, and selenium actually contribute to mental clarity. Vitamin B helps brain neurotransmitters reduce cognitive decline, thus improving focus and memory; vitamin B_2 (riboflavin) boosts energy and metabolism. Iron enhances brain activity.

The following vitamins promote clarity and memory as well as overall physical health and weight loss:

- Vitamin C: kiwi, peppers, oranges, tomatoes, papaya, mango, zucchini

- Vitamin E: whole grains, nuts, tomatoes, spinach, broccoli, fish, onions

- Calcium: low-fat dairy products, sesame seeds, tofu, white beans, bok choy

- B vitamins: turkey, tuna, whole grains, lentils, beans

- Selenium: Brazil nuts, tuna, shellfish, cashews, eggs, lentils, sunflower seeds

- Iron: beef, chicken, almonds, and quinoa (pronounced *keen-wah*, a rice-like food with a rich, nutty taste that is often considered a grain but is actually a seed

By making simple enhancements to our daily food intake, we can choose to enrich our current diets with foods that promote energy, clarity, and overall better brain function! For example, a mango salsa is a tasty addition to any salad, sandwich, or even an omelet. Clear your mind even more by keeping chopped spinach, onions, and tomatoes on hand to create a topping for chicken, enjoy as a side salad, or add to a wrap. Squeeze some lime juice on edamame for a light and refreshing snack. Sprinkle sesame seeds onto your pasta or in a salad. Add beans to your brownie mix, make quinoa with pine nuts as a quick and tasty side dish.

Ricotta and scrambled eggs make for a simple, healthy, delicious brain dump brunch.

Fluffy, Light Ricotta and Scrambled Eggs with Zucchini Hash Browns

Jazz up scrambled eggs and pack them with the clarity-boosting nutrients mentioned above. It takes less than fifteen minutes to prepare and is filled with flavor, textures, and lots of health benefits.

Serves 1.

What You'll Need
2 eggs
¼ cup part-skim ricotta cheese
sea salt
freshly ground pepper
1 tomato, chopped (optional)
1 zucchini, shredded
¼ onion, chopped
olive oil spray

Let's Do This
Mix together the eggs, ricotta, salt, and pepper. For a little extra pizzazz, I like to add a chopped tomato, but you can include whatever veggies you like. Cook them as you would your favorite scrambled eggs.

To make the zucchini hash browns, combine the zucchini and onion and cook in a hot skillet sprayed with olive oil until browned. Flip and brown the other side. You can drain the liquid and form them into patties if you'd like, or just keep them loose.

Center Your Focus

Don't ask what the world needs. Ask what makes
you come alive, and go do it. Because what the
world needs is people who have come alive.

—Howard Thurman

When I was in eighth grade, I was chosen as one of four speakers to give the eighth-grade commencement speech. I was at the podium in my cap and gown describing what it was like to feel like you don't fit in. I told the crowd about my first day of kindergarten. My mother had dressed me in a green plaid kilt with knee-high socks and a cardigan sweater. I was the tallest kid in the class. So tall, I didn't even fit in the desk. "There I stood, Jolly Green Jennifer," I detailed my experience to an auditorium filled with proud parents, aunts, and uncles. I spoke about the power of kindness, that we shouldn't judge each other because of our differences and flaws, and then I even talked about believing in our dreams.

After I finished, the crowd applauded. Many people came up to me to share their own stories of not fitting in. Others shared dreams they had for the future. I was only thirteen, but I felt on top of the world speaking and sharing a bit of myself that day! Recalling it now, it feels like yesterday, but for a long while, I forgot about that little girl. I didn't remember that I inspired people, that I had a voice, that I had something to share. Instead, I hid in the corner of a room under a mane of hair practically covering my face.

I made a friend, though, who really liked and accepted me exactly as I was. She didn't see the unworthy girl I saw when I looked in the mirror. She saw the real me, the me who had dreams, loved to help others, and liked to share silly stories. In talking with her, I opened up about myself. She asked me questions about my childhood, happy memories, and fun times, and the eighth-grade graduation speech came up in conversation. The memory of that day, the feeling I got from writing and sharing and inspiring, suddenly came back to me and allowed me to believe in myself again.

Brain dumping serves several purposes. We've discussed the importance of releasing what's on your mind to make space for present-moment energy. Now we will move from **brain dumping to release** to **brain dumping to believe.**

In order to do this, I'll guide you through the process of defining your core values. Next I'll show you the importance of learning from your own positive life experiences and rekindling your power of creativity and imagination. Then I'll help you create a revived life vision.

But first you have to work on believing in yourself. Self-belief is like a muscle—you have to work it to keep it strong. It's so much easier to believe in yourself when you are in touch with who you really are, when you are aware of your strengths, gifts, and talents, *and* when you are using them regularly to serve the world.

In this part of the chapter, we are going to adjust your focus to shine a light on your core values and your individual strengths—what you *can* do, what you *can* control. We'll elicit self-discovery through brain dumping about positive past experiences.

When I meet with women, I expect greatness from them—that they will do whatever it is they set out to do. I expect that they will succeed. There's no doubt in my mind. If it's in their hearts to do something, create something, achieve something, I know they can and they will.

I know you have the power to do the same thing—to truly transform from the inside out. I wouldn't be writing this book if I didn't believe every single one of us can do this. I expect greatness from you. I have no doubt in my mind that you are a complete, whole, capable, incredibly strong and talented human being who can and will create whatever you want for your life.

I want you to expect greatness from yourself too. You are valuable, beautiful, and worthwhile, and you can achieve whatever you commit to, anything that is in your heart.

Zen Quickie

Visualize Joy

Spend half a minute seeing yourself joyful. The visualization should not only include the way you look, but also your vitality, energy, and attitude. Use your imagination to envision all the good things in life. Feel your heart beating strong, your blood sugar stabilizing, and your body utilizing food as fuel and digesting well. Envision healthy relationships at home, at work, with your friends and family. Visualize yourself smiling, laughing, and jumping for joy.

Knowing Your Worth and Defining Your Values

Each of us has a core value system. Our values are the internal compass that guide us through life and anchor us in turbulent times. All the choices you make, down to the food you put in your body, express your values. Knowing, honoring, and living by your core values is a key factor in motivating lasting behavior change.

Overstuffed schedules and stress can cause an (unintentional) lack of focus on what really matters. This lack of focus can disconnect us from our core values. Without an internal compass, we begin attaching our self-worth to things or circumstances, and then we are motivated by those rather than our true values. I was speaking with a dear friend recently, and we were talking about this very subject. Too many of us attach our value to things outside ourselves rather than honoring our inherent worth as humans.

I have two children, LuLu and the Little Man. They are precious, with imaginations that run wild. We play, we hop around the house like frogs, and we imagine a café in our backyard where we hold socials for all our imaginary friends. I could never look at my children and attach their worth to anything.

Why is it so difficult to look in the mirror and do the same thing for ourselves?

We are all worthy. No strings attached. *You are worthy.*

I know this is a difficult concept to grasp, because we constantly attach strings to our worth—the number on the scale, the money in a bank account, the number of clients on a roster, or the opinions of others. Many women feel worthless because they are overweight, in debt, or not achieving the goals they set for themselves years ago.

All these strings can affect our worth, which in turn affects everything else. A mom may be so wrapped up in her children that she ties her self-worth to their successes. A woman may be so glued to her career that she doesn't even know who she is without it. And so many of us connect our self-worth to ridiculous expectations of perfection, and when we fall short we run for food or shoe shopping or even pills to numb us from feelings of disappointment . . . self-worth can be a tangled mess when we attach strings to it.

The thing is, our essence—who we are each born to be—is not attached to anything. No matter what situation our experience throws at us, no matter what test we are given, we still are worthy. Even when we don't feel like it, even when we want to crawl in a cave and hibernate, we are each a whole, complete, capable, resourceful, and talented person. But often that picture gets muddled because we focus too much on outcomes: losing weight, getting a promotion, opening a business, getting approval, winning recognition, or earning love . . . the list goes on. Thinking about outcomes affects the paths we take. For example, in my twenties I would sometimes think, *If I wear this outfit, then tonight I will probably meet someone.* Little did I know, my future husband would fall in love with me while I was wearing baggy old sweats and my hair was tied in a knot on top of my head.

We must delve deeper than outcome and instead do what stirs the soul, serves others, and allows us to use our unique gifts to help the world. When we simply use our gifts, people flow into our lives, doors open, and experiences happen that are even bigger than we could have imagined.

I learned I was worthy without strings attached by letting go of almost every concept I believed could affect my worth. After experiencing some financial issues a few years ago, my husband and I sold our home, turned in our vehicle, auctioned off our china, and shed many of the possessions that typically define people. I remember sobbing while my baby Lu napped. I prayed to God for an answer, and He told me to write. Writing is something I've done practically since birth. But for some reason, I didn't even feel worthy of picking up my pen at that time.

Grabbing whatever scrap piece of paper I could find, I started jotting down my thoughts. In that moment, I realized God was telling me it would be all right and that I should carry on and continue the work I was doing. We must use our gifts to serve the world. After that, a whole new chapter emerged. I felt peace that no possession or outcome could ever deliver. It was like the intense love I feel when I hold my children, kiss my husband, see a baby giggle, have a heart-to-heart with my mom, spend time with my dad, or witness a person truly smiling. That peace stayed with me, and I remembered my core values and that faith was my anchor as well as my compass—and that I am worthy (no strings attached).

Every single person, regardless of circumstance, history, race, color, religion—every one of us is worthy. Find your anchor and compass in your core values, and you will free yourself from the strings that you are attaching to your worth.

What's Your Operating System?

When you operate without honoring your core values, you lose direction; then you look to others for the magic solution when you really have all the answers you need within yourself. To find them, you have to be still, reconnect, and listen.

By reconnecting with your core values, you discover your best self, the magnificent woman you were born to be. You put your values in motion, consciously make an effort to express your values, set goals with your values in mind, and reignite your spark for life.

When you are fully connected to your core values, you find it much easier to let go of behaviors that don't serve you. You create a life free of attachments (to outcomes, possessions, or people) and addictions. You release fear, ignite your spirit, and use your gifts and talents to serve the world. You set value-based standards of behaviors for yourself and others.

TAKE ACTION

. . . .

IDENTIFY YOUR CORE VALUES

Using the list below (and adding any of your own), pick four to six of your most important core values. Be authentic—choose not what you think you should value, but what is in your soul. A value is not something you should be guilted into—it is who you are.

You may hold a number of the values listed below. Remember, too, that our priorities change as we travel through different seasons of our lives. But by honing in on the four to six that resonate most with you *in this moment*, you will begin to give yourself, your life, and your well-being direction and meaning.

After you've identified your core values, write them down in your B.A.L.A.N.C.E. Journal because we will refer back to them later in the book.

abundance, achievement, acknowledgment, altruism, appreciation, authenticity, autonomy, beauty, belonging, bravery, camaraderie, candor, certainty, choice, collaboration, comfort, community, compassion, contribution, creativity, decorum, directness, discovery, dreaming, drive, education, excellence, exploring, faith, fame, family, fascination, flexibility, flow, fluency, freedom, friendship, generosity, grace, growth, guidance, happiness, harmony, health, holiness, honesty, hopefulness, humor, imagination, independence, industry, joy, justice, keenness, kindness, leadership, learning, liberation, loyalty, maturity, modesty, nerve, optimism, order, passion, philanthropy, playfulness, precision, privacy, respect, security, self-expression, service, solitude, speed, spirituality, thankfulness, tolerance, tradition, trust, understanding, usefulness, warmth, wisdom, youth, zeal

For a more extensive values list, check out my website Inspirista Lifestyle and the Inspired Girl blog (http://inspiredgirl.net/list-of-values). You can also work with a coach trained in values programs.

. . . .

Learn from Your Experiences

It's kind of funny, but for some people it's easier to recall and retell bad experiences than good ones. A friend may not call you to tell you about the gorgeous bird she saw while getting into her car, but if a bird pooped on her head, you'd hear all about it.

What's more, we are hard on ourselves. Women do absolutely extraordinary things all the time, but we often don't see ourselves as extraordinary. We focus on our failures rather than on our successes.

It's time to refocus that negative lens and begin thinking about positive perspectives.

TAKE ACTION

OPEN UP TO YOUR OWN WISDOM

This exercise will help you learn from yourself and your experiences. Consider each of the following calls to action. You may even want to write your thoughts in your B.A.L.A.N.C.E. Journal.

1. **Spotlight yourself.** Think about you as your best self, when you are fully engaged and plugged in to life. You may remember a specific situation or an overall feeling. Envision it in a way that brings it back clearly and vividly for you.

2. **Recall an engaging experience.** What was your most powerful experience with your life, your health, your body, your self-esteem—a time when you felt most alive? What made it so energizing? Who was there? What surrounded you? Describe the specific experience in detail.

3. **Focus on what's working.** Identify areas of your life that are working well. Describe clear examples of past and present outcomes that you deem a success.

4. **Identify your strengths.** Women are amazingly strong. We juggle many things without even flinching. We help others without question. List some of your strengths and describe them in full detail.

5. **Unleash your can-do attitude.** Forget limitations. Let go of what you *can't* do. Challenge yourself to think in terms of what's possible, and what you *can* do. Acknowledge all you can do, all you can control, and don't give power to what you can't. Make a list of things you can start doing *now* to be your healthiest self.

It's hard to separate your self-worth from your experiences. But experiences can be out of your control, so you must separate them from yourself. You are not your experiences. You can use them to fuel a fire for the greater good, to teach yourself something, or to teach others. But don't let them define you or your worth. Some of the most amazing achievements in history came in response to tragedy. Instead of being broken by disease or financial upheaval or unemployment or loss, take energy from those experiences and use them as a catalyst for change.

Rekindle Your Power to Create

I remember once after a quick trip to the dollar store, my kids and I came home with modeling clay. We opened the box and got right to work on creating shapes. My son wanted to make a snowman with a hat, and my daughter set out to create an ice-cream cone with a cherry on top. Next we made a family, then a flower, a basketball, a birthday cake, and the alphabet. We molded and messed up and started again and mixed colors and created for hours on end. It was a blast.

Playing with modeling clay made me think how gratifying it is to create something. There's a joy that we get when we start from scratch—the song writer creating music, the builder constructing a home, the farmer growing vegetables, the artist molding a sculpture. I find more joy in baking a cake with eggs, flour, and sugar than with a box mix.

The modeling clay also made me think about the power we each have to create something out of nothing. Look at the highways where once there were dirt roads and, before that, just land. It is incredible. We all have that power, each with our own talents. When we combine our unique gifts with the power we have to create something, the sky really is the limit.

I always say limitless possibilities emerge with creativity and imagination. We are all born with this ability, but sometimes as we get older, our creativity is suppressed or we're taught to fit a mold that doesn't allow for imagination. And then we forget what makes us come alive.

It is so important, though, to question ourselves so we remember what our gifts are and so we use them to serve the world. I've witnessed the power of imagination and creativity in my own life as well as in the lives of many of my friends, family members, and clients. This is key to being filled with passion and energy, to being our healthiest, happiest selves.

I am a volunteer for the nonprofit organization Enchanted Makeovers (EM). The importance of passion is one of the many reasons why EM's work is so significant and so very close to my heart. Terry Grahl, EM's founder and chief visionary, is a true kindred spirit. She sees the possibilities, and EM transforms physical shelter spaces into whimsical cottage retreat centers where the women and children can thrive, where dreams and hope can live.

Every one of us—whether volunteer, investor, or woman or child living in the shelter—every single one of us experiences the sheer power of the imagination. It allows us to each have our own internal enchanted makeover.

As you travel on your balance journey, think about rekindling your dormant creativity and imagination. Think about ways you can be creative and express your talents. How can you be creative even in areas where you think you have no talent? Even if you can't draw a straight line, you may still have fun sketching or painting. Once you let go of feelings of limitation, fear, and worry, there's no end to what you can create.

Create Your Revived Life Vision

Without leaps of imagination, or dreaming, we lose the excitement of possibilities. Dreaming, after all, is a form of planning.

—Gloria Steinem

Vision. This is one of the most common elements for actualization of our dreams. Vision allows you to see clearly from your heart into your mind's eye, watching it like a movie. Vision is what guides you beyond the past and moving toward the future.

Tucked away in each of us is a dream, a purpose, something we were born to do to serve the world. But in order to dream while we are awake, we must revive our life vision, really look within, take the dream out of hiding, and give it power by visualizing it in living color.

Creating a revived vision for yourself is the foundation to making *any* kind of change in your life. If you don't have a vision, you won't know where you're going—it's like planning to meet a dear friend for lunch without knowing exactly where she is waiting for you. You may never find her. To better understand yourself, you need to take some time to uncover truths that you may have forgotten. Careful questioning helps you discover who you are and what you want.

Don't worry, I haven't forgotten that you really, *really* want to release weight off of your body. Remember that the best way to balance your weight is to live your life in balance. And the best way to do that is to create a revived life vision that extends way beyond numbers on a scale. I've seen this time and time again. When women focus on creating a healthy vision, sustained weight loss happens naturally. When weight loss is the only goal, it is a temporary change that leads to a lifetime of getting on and off the Dieting Wheel of Frustration.

To create your vision, you have to really see who and what you were born to be. You have to look into your heart and use your mind's eye to visualize what being healthy really looks like. You have to feel it with every fiber of your being. You have to see it so much that you believe it is happening now.

Many women laugh when I first describe the concept of vision. One woman even shouted during class, "I just want to see myself thinner!"

I heard her loud and clear, so I asked the group, "If I waved a magic wand, and *poof* you were thinner, would the weight loss alone really make you feel happy and fulfilled?" Of course, their answer was a resounding no.

From my personal experience (and having worked with women of every shape and size), I know that weight loss does not equate to joy, health, happiness, fulfillment, or success. Success on the scale does not mean success in life. As a matter of fact, I can't define what success in life means to you. Only you can determine that for yourself. I've chased the holy grail of a size 4, I've been there, but when I got there, I chased for the holy grail of a boyfriend, the holy grail of a pair of shoes, the holy grail of a career. Chasing for external happiness was just that: a never-ending chase. I set out to explore what truly can create a life of joy, health, happiness, and balance . . . and my conclusion was simply this: It lies within ourselves. It begins with love of self and with vision, faith, intention, and purposeful action. We all can—and you *will*—create whatever you truly want and deserve for your life, including releasing the weight (off your mind, off your shoulders, and off your body) you are holding on to.

So if your vision is simply a thinner version of the current you, keep looking. See yourself living the best version of your life possible as a passionate, vibrant version of yourself. Steps and goals are all well and good, but if you're not pulling your vision from a deep, personal place, the steps will get you nowhere. I believe the vision often lends itself to creating the steps naturally, and it doesn't feel like exhausting work, but rather an exciting movement forward.

Creating your revived life vision can take some persistence, as Sasha found. At first, her vision was narrow—she simply wanted to weigh less. But when she pushed herself to really picture what she wanted, here's what she told me: "I see myself happy, openly dancing with my husband. I see myself playing games with my kids and not getting winded. I see myself having the energy to go for long walks with my best friend and having confidence to stand in front of a room full of people to give a great presentation at work. I see myself strong and smiling."

Now *that* is a vision!

Studies show that 86 percent of women feel most beautiful when they are fulfilled and happy in their lives. My guess is that you don't simply want to lose weight. You want to feel excited to be alive. You want to feel great about getting up in the morning, taking care of your family, going to work, spending time with good friends, having fun, being creative, and glowing with emotional, physical, and spiritual health. You want to have the energy to do things that bring joy and happiness.

TAKE ACTION

CREATE A VISION STATEMENT FOR YOUR LIFE

To do this, you must release all boundaries, obstacles, fears, and limiting beliefs from your mind. Without limitation, close your eyes and see a detailed vision for your life. Picture yourself, your attitude, your temper, your demeanor. Hear yourself speak. Watch yourself move. What is your life like? Describe your relationships, your home, your family life, your career, your fun. Be as detailed and specific as possible. Have fun. Imagine moments. Use your talents. Help others with them. See yourself at work—contributing, being heard, sharing. Picture your body in motion and working to its full capacity, pushing yourself beyond your comfort zone. Imagine food as your energizer and feel yourself enjoying the taste, texture, and flavor of natural, fresh, vibrantly colored foods. Imagine yourself living a life that is in full balance with your core values.

In your B.A.L.A.N.C.E. Journal, describe your vision statement in full detail. I strongly believe that we must be the cocreator of our lives, and that means knowing exactly how we want our lives to look, feel, and be. It's empowering to take the driver's seat and live on purpose.

This activity isn't very structured. It's kind of your free space to bust open your dream and let it out. Ideally you'll be smiling the whole time during this activity because your life vision should make you happy. If it stresses you out, it's not the right life vision for you.

Here are some other ways to think about your life vision:

Find a quiet space so you can dream while awake. This is an incredible experience (and a blast too!). It allows you to release all boundaries, walls, and obstacles. Picture in color and motion what you are doing. Begin with your personal life—family, home life, the way your space is decorated, the things you do for fun, what you are passionate about, how you maintain an active lifestyle. Next, move into your career or professional life. Picture your office space, see what you are doing, and feel the positive impact you are making.

Remember, we are acting *as if.* We are not worrying about *the how*—it does not matter right now. There are no boundaries. No rules. You are defining your success. What is your overall philosophy on life?

Key note: Dreaming while you are awake is not about daydreaming. Remember, there are certain nonnegotiables in your life, and if you are daydreaming about something that simply cannot happen because of one of your nonnegotiables, you are wasting your energy, and you'll always feel unfilled. Make sure your dream aligns with your core values.

Next: Imagine that anything you desire has come to be and that you are living exactly the life you've envisioned.

Create a vision collage. Using a board, wall, box, book, or space of any kind (digital or physical) start to gather images of anything and everything you find pleasing—anything you want to achieve or have as part of your life. Be creative! You can clip photos or words out of magazines and newspapers, take photographs, or find color swatches of paint. Because we are whole people, it's important to notice what you like as it pertains to life in general, not just specifically to weight loss.

When Margie did this for the first time, she was a bit discouraged. She said, "Jenn, I don't think my vision board is very good. It seems kind of shallow—it just looks pretty, but there's no real substance to it yet." I looked at her board, which was, in fact, absolutely gorgeous. There was a string of pearls on it, lace trimmings, beautiful flowers. I questioned her about why she chose certain items, and she wasn't sure. We talked a bit more, and Margie (who works as an office manager) told me she always wished she did something with decorating people's homes. It was a natural gift; every time I stepped into her bathroom I felt like I was at a beautiful country cottage retreat center. The aha moment came to us—Margie's board wasn't shallow at all; it was a vision that she wanted to do more decorating, helping people create beautiful, meaningful homes.

If Margie hadn't created the board, she wouldn't have been able to see what she was feeling. She sent away for a class registration schedule to begin a home decorating business. Even if it begins as a hobby or part-time endeavor, Margie said she would feel fulfilled. And she recognizes that when she's fulfilled in spirit, she is not as hungry for unnecessary filler food to fill her up.

You can turn your dreaming into a written vision statement, you can paste pictures in your journal and scrapbook your vision, or you can use a large board—the most important part is that you have a visual or written reminder of the vision that you just created in your mind.

Create a Vision Book

If you like something tangible but the idea of a vision collage, board, or wall seems a little hokey, grab your favorite notebook or journal and begin a vision book. Inspirista Angela Jia Kim, founder of Om Aroma & Co. and Savor the Success, is amazing at creating what she wants for her life, and she has helped women around the world do the same. She suggests documenting everything you want to happen in your personal and professional life in one vision book. She uses her vision book as a means not only to visualize but also to design (in words) the steps to make the vision come to be. She says a vision book should be a specific and detailed blueprint—not someone else's, but your own. Your vision book helps move your imagination to the physical world. Angela begins by using pictures or sketches, and then as she is inspired, she writes the related action next to it. Angela says, "The more clear you are, the more you can manifest what you want!"

Here are Angela Jia Kim's four steps to creating a vision book of your own:

1. **Scratch it out on paper.** Do a brain dump. It's okay if it's messy. This is your chance to get thoughts out and experiment with words and ideas, even though they may not be perfect. Just get it out without worrying about perfection. Use interesting paper that you already have—it's metaphoric for using what you have to get what you want. Recycled paper, receipts, a child's painting, and note cards are all fantastic pieces to use. We often have so many experiences and current assets that we don't use but that can catapult us to the next level. Use what you have!

2. **Refine.** Ask for advice. After you are somewhat clear on your vision, find coaches, mentors, or people who have done some-

thing similar, and reach out for help. Take the advice you like and refine the plan to suit you and your life.

3. **Pull out to-dos and next steps.** Assign them to someone or to yourself. Put them in your calendar.

4. **Get a support team.** They'll help you and hold you accountable.

Make and sign a commitment contract to yourself. Make a contract with yourself and commit to your vision statement or vision collage by writing a very simple one-line commitment pledge and signing off on it. You deserve to live the best version of your life possible, so commit to it! For example:

> *I am committed to being present in my life, to being an active participant in my life, to taking footsteps toward the dream that is in my heart, to living on purpose, and to holding strong to my*

B.A.L.A.N.C.E. Tip

Don't Wait for Change

Push yourself to do something now. Walk that trail, ride that bike, swim in the ocean, run a race, buy a new dress and salsa dance. Don't wait for change to happen. We've all said, "When I am thinner, when I am healthier, I will. . . ." But remember, we are complete, capable, and perfect as we are today; we just have to believe in ourselves, and then we can achieve anything. See yourself as healthy and balanced today, and you *will be* healthy and balanced. We live up to our own expectations of ourselves, so set the bar high and soar!

vision. I commit to living a healthy life, to nurturing my body as it is an instrument to using my gifts to serve the world, and to being a healthy example for everyone I care about in my life.

Congratulations!

You have created a revived life vision and have made a firm commitment to change your life. You're one giant leap closer to finding balance from within, transforming your life, and shedding that which weighs you down.

Everyday B.A.L.A.N.C.E. Technique: *Breathe*

There are times when no matter how calm you try to be, no matter how much you brain dump, your mind still swirls. You will be busy, frantic, running, concerned, worried, and stressed. This is life, we are human, and it happens. There will be situations we cannot control. We will make mistakes. We will fail.

Even during the most chaotic, stressful times in your life, you can use simple tools to help clear your mind and feel lighter and calmer.

I identified these Everyday B.A.L.A.N.C.E. Techniques while dealing with my own very personal, very difficult situations. During those times, stress began to pile up, along with some of the weight I had worked so hard to release years before. I was struggling to get healthy again, to get back to balance. And then I had a lightbulb moment: balance isn't *getting*, it's *being*. I took a deep breath, and then another. Breathing in and out, slowly and mindfully, I let go of regrets about the past and apprehension about the future. That moment was pure light. I loved the way it felt. I gave myself permission just to *be* by breathing.

Everyone breathes—we die if we don't. But most of us don't breathe properly. We take shallow breaths and take in just enough oxygen to get by. That's automatic breathing. Add mindfulness, and breathing delivers so much more.

Mindful breathing is deep. When you breathe deeply, you send extra oxygen to your brain and the cells of your body. Actual biochemical changes occur in your body right away. You feel more relaxed because your body immediately begins to produce lower levels of the stress hormones, such as cortisol, that rev you up and can make you feel nervous. Mindful breathing can lower your heart rate, blood pressure, and muscle tension; boost your mood by reducing anxiety and feelings of depression; and facilitate healthy digestion.

Begin to notice the way you breathe. Like many of my clients, you'll probably notice that you hold your breath a lot. Yawning, sighing, and feelings of fogginess and fatigue are signs that you're not getting enough oxygen.

TAKE ACTION

. . . .

PRACTICE MINDFUL BREATHING

Mindful breathing—also known as diaphragmatic breathing or belly breathing—is a skill that you can learn with a bit of practice. Over time, it can become second nature. Here's how to do it:

1. **Inhale deeply and slowly through your nose.** As you inhale, allow your lungs to fill and your belly to expand to make room for all the air you're taking in. Hold the air in your lungs for a few seconds to give your lungs time to absorb oxygen and to let your body relax.

2. **Slowly exhale through your mouth.** Use your abdominal muscles to help your diaphragm push the air out of your chest.

3. **Repeat several times.**

Practice mindful breathing a few times a day—when you get up, while you're stopped at traffic lights, before you go to bed, and so on.

And whenever you're feeling stressed, overwhelmed, anxious, worried, or upset, take a few moments to breathe mindfully. You will soon feel calmer and better able to cope with whatever is bothering you.

. . . .

Summing Up

In this chapter, we've discussed the benefits of brain dumping as well as some great ways to empty your mind of clutter. We've also looked at the benefits of breathing deeply and mindfully. The activities I suggested include:

- Do a free-form brain dump to move worrisome thoughts from your brain to your B.A.L.A.N.C.E. Journal.

- Do an exercise that will help you center your focus on your strengths, your abilities, and your past successes to discover your strongest self.

- Use what you've learned in your brain dump to create a revived life vision and a vision statement for your life.

- Eat mind-clarifying foods that are rich sources of vitamin C, vitamin E, B vitamins, and iron.

- Practice deep breathing, which reduces feelings of stress and calms your anxious mind.

In Chapter 3, I'll share some assessment tools that will help you look honestly and completely at your life as it is now so you'll have the knowledge you need to move toward where you want to be.

Chapter Three

. . . .

A is for
Assess and Accept

I think self-awareness is probably the most
important thing towards being a champion.

—Billie Jean King

. . . .

Once when I was driving to an event in an unfamiliar neighborhood, I thought I knew where I was going, but it seemed
like I had been driving in circles for twenty minutes. Finally
I called the venue to ask for directions. I told them I was a bit lost, so
naturally the first question they asked me was, "Where are you now?"
I looked at a street sign and told them the name, but I didn't know
if I was north- or southbound on the street, I wasn't even sure what
town I was in, and I couldn't identify a landmark because I was in a
residential neighborhood.

The woman on the phone couldn't help me. "I'm sorry, dear. I can't
tell you where to go if you don't know where you are. Find out and call
me back."

The same is true for life. Living and knowing the truth of who you are in this moment, and assessing and accepting the woman you are, opens you up to being the woman you were born to be.

When I was younger, I had a hard time with this, especially with facing my own body, so I often ignored it. I avoided mirrors, tore myself out of pictures, and would never let someone with a measuring tape near me. I think I probably did that with many aspects in my life—I swept details under the rug until one day the lump under the carpet was so big, I couldn't help but trip over it.

Why was I so judgmental of my own circumstances, my own body? I remember deciding to make peace with the mirror. Taking the blindfold off opened my eyes to who I was and where I was, and by assessing and accepting that woman and her position, I was on the path to restoring myself and my self-esteem. I may not have been nurturing my body as well as I could have been, but I had a core belief system that, with a little attention, could be strong and guide me through life in a deeper way than I had been allowing. Those values would bring me back to a place of loving myself. I had talents I wasn't utilizing, but with a little dusting off, I could bring them back to life so I could live with passion and energy and so I could serve a purpose, no matter how big or small it may have been. Continually facing my truth allows me to stretch and grow to reach my full potential, and I am sure as you face yours, you will feel the same way.

I definitely relate to women when they first come in to Curves and say they don't want to be measured or fill out a current-state analysis when they begin coaching. I don't push, but I do share my own story, and it usually opens them up to assessing and accepting themselves too.

In this chapter, I'll help you assess your life as it is now so you'll have the information you need to plan where you want to go and how to get there.

Looking at Now

Assessing is all about self-discovery, about taking a clear, honest look at your current situation and your true self in order to create a lasting, effective personal transformation plan. Your plan must align with who you are as a person, your core values, and what's important in your life. If these aspects aren't factored in, you will feel like you are *doing* rather than *being*—just going through the motions rather than actually living a healthy life that aligns with your unique personality.

In order to create and reach your goals, you've got to take an introspective look at who you are and what you truly value, meanwhile rediscovering who you were born to be. Accepting your own reality and understanding that true transformation takes work (and personal responsibility) are key to moving forward.

So to find balance in life and with the scale, assess these key areas:

1. **Your body**—including your strength, physical structure, health, and physical energy source (food)

2. **Your internal muscle**—including your core values and mental energy source (attitude)

3. **Your caring balance**—the delicate balance of how you care for others vs. how you care for yourself

4. **Your schedule**—including your lifestyle factors and the way you use time, because the busyness of your life can have a huge impact on your ability to be in balance

The Balanced Inspirista graphic on the following page shows you in a nutshell what we'll be assessing. Don't worry if it doesn't make a lot of sense right now—it will soon.

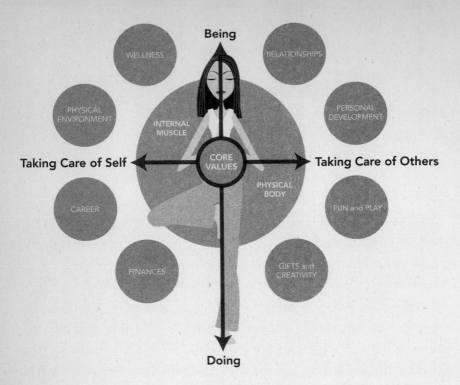

- In the center, you'll notice are the **core values.** As we discussed in Chapter 2, these will serve as your anchor to keep you centered regardless of life circumstances as well as your compass to guide you through life.

- Your **physical body** and your **internal muscle** combined create your overall strength. Having strength creates the confidence necessary to move forward with your vision, believe in yourself, and use your gifts to serve the world.

- Your **lifestyle** factors create your schedule. An overall sense of being in balance combines your **overall strength** with your **lifestyle factors** and **caring balance.**

In your B.A.L.A.N.C.E. Journal, create an **Assessment** that looks like this:

Body	Strength	Health	Internal Muscle	Priorities	Delegating

What's Your Success Scale?

How do you measure success? By the numbers on the scale? How your jeans fit? How much energy you feel? How much food you eat? How much you've exercised? What people say about you?

It's important to understand how you view success because you may be judging yourself in ways that are destructive or that no longer work for you. If your expectations are not realistic, you can change them. You want your success scale to motivate you to continue healthy behaviors, not to punish you when you fall short of perfection.

Some people are motivated by numbers. "Seeing my weight go down motivates me to continue being healthy," says Margie. And it's true for Margie—she lost over forty pounds in our first few months working together, and she is making very healthy food choices.

Other people prefer less concrete measures of success; watching the numbers on the scale drains them. Denise recently said almost the exact opposite of Margie. We weighed her weekly, and even though she continually lost weight, she didn't want to know the number. "Jennifer, I've lost weight before, and when I was motivated by the number on the scale, I would do just about anything to get it down, even to the detriment of my health. I just want to know that I feel good and that I am making healthy choices. Just seeing salad and fruit in my refrigerator is success to me."

Assessing Your Body

How do you feel about your body? Back when my self-image was completely out of balance, I went out of my way to avoid mirrors and photos of myself. I didn't like my body, and the less I had to look at it, the better. But once I learned to love and accept myself, my appreciation for my body deepened. Taking the very important first step of assessing and accepting my body paved the way for me to nurture it in a variety of healthy ways.

At Curves, when we meet with potential members for the first time, we do a complimentary figure analysis. This analysis includes a full-body assessment, measuring body size, body fat, body mass index, and weight as well as identifying places of pain, discomfort, and weakness. We test cardiovascular endurance, muscle strength, and flexibility. This figure analysis is so important because many women do not have an accurate, current assessment of their own bodies. We have to develop a relationship with ourselves, and doing a figure analysis is kind of like a first date—we are getting to know ourselves. I can't tell you how many women don't know their measurements, haven't looked in a full-length mirror in years, and simply have no clue about their cardiovascular or muscular endurance. The first step toward change is recognizing, acknowledging, and accepting what *is*—then we are ready to take ourselves to the next level and move forward.

As opposed to being critical of your body, assessment is a means to grow deeper in gratitude for your body. Often when a woman completes a body assessment or figure analysis, she is amazed and inspired by her own strength. By assessing your body, you are actually reconnecting with it!

Do You See What I See?

On a piece of paper, draw your shape the way you see it in your mind. Then, in a form-fitting outfit, take a full-length photograph and compare the shape you drew with the shape in the photo—it's amazing to compare the shape you see in your mind's eye to what actually is.

You may break out in a cold sweat at the thought of being photographed in Spandex. But it's actually a wonderful exercise because it allows you to start releasing judgment and accepting your body as it is in the present moment. Accepting is a precursor to self-love and self-nurturing.

Believe it or not, I find that most women do not see themselves the way they actually are or as others see them, and they generally have a very skewed self-image. They nitpick and focus on what they think are the flawed areas rather than the overall image of the beautiful, unique, amazing women that others see. So in this very important assessment, they can look at a photograph in order to learn to accept and appreciate themselves as they are at that moment. I can't tell you how many women have not looked at themselves in a full-length mirror in years because they can't stand the image staring back at them. How can you possibly love and nurture a woman you won't even face? But I understand—I was that woman too.

If you're ready for the Spandex, take a picture and focus on your beauty. Notice your curves, honor them. Look at the shape of your eyes, the beautiful color of your hair, the softness of your skin, the length of your neck, and the warmth in your smile. Connect with the woman in the photo and see her as your best friend.

TAKE ACTION

. . . .

DO YOUR OWN BODY ASSESSMENT

In your B.A.L.A.N.C.E. Journal, create a page that looks like this (or go to your local Curves and have a complimentary figure analysis):

Date: _____

Measurements:

    Chest/Back _____

    Waist _____

    Abdomen _____

    Hips _____

    Thighs _____

    Arms _____

    Calves _____

Weight:

    Time _____

    Weight _____

    Clothing _____

Pain Issues:

    Where _____

    How Often _____

    Intensity _____

10-second heart rate:

    Resting _____

       (beats of your pulse when you are sitting still)

    Active _____

       (beats of your pulse after doing 30 seconds of jumping jacks)

Here's a sample from Lesley's B.A.L.A.N.C.E. Journal:

Date: 8/1/11

Measurements:

Chest/Back	47
Waist	36¼
Abdomen	45½
Hips	52
Thighs	31
Arms	16¼
Calves	15½

Weight:

Time	7 A.M.
Weight	267
Clothing	Birthday Suit

Pain Issues:

Where	Feet, Back
How Often	Daily, especially when sitting for long periods of time
Intensity	Varies, usually Tylenol helps

10-second heart rate:

Resting	13
Active	24 (and VERY winded!!)

• •

Assessing Your Health

I know having borderline diabetes was certainly my wake-up call, and many clients come to me when they feel their health is at risk. If you haven't had a full physical lately, now is a good time to make an appointment so you can find out your current blood pressure, blood sugar, cholesterol levels, and so forth.

Be honest with yourself and your doctor about any health symptoms, early warning signs, or risk factors. If you have a family history of heart disease, diabetes, high cholesterol, or cancer, make a note of it. Preparing a list of these risks as well as your questions for your doctor is the best way to get the most out of your appointment. Knowing your current state of health will help you when you are figuring out the healthiest food choices for you. You have the power to overcome many health problems by changing your lifestyle.

Assessing Your Diet

A few years back, my cousin bought a tank of bargain gas at a service station that he'd never been to before. An hour later, his car broke down; the guys at the garage said the gasoline had been watered down. It cost him a thousand dollars to fix the damage. Now he fuels his car with only high-quality gas from trusted stations.

Not taking good care of our possessions can cause costly problems. We know this. Yet with our most valuable possession—our body—we are often careless. We fuel it with drive-through junk and vending-machine mystery food containing ingredients we can't even pronounce. Then we wonder why we hit the wall by mid-afternoon, depleted and empty.

The type of fuel we take in affects everything we do, say, think, and feel. Low-quality food breaks us down, and high-quality food helps us to be the best version of ourselves possible. It's just like fueling up the car's tank: low-quality gas breaks down the engine, but good fuel keeps it running smoothly.

In the following section, we'll assess the foods you use for fuel and identify their effect on your mind and body.

TAKE ACTION

· ·

WHAT'S YOUR FOOD-MOOD CONNECTION?

Food can have a profound effect on your mood and your attitude. It causes a chemical reaction that can make you feel happy or sad, connected or distant, tired or energized. Certain foods can amplify feelings of anxiety and stress; others can calm you. They can also affect your brain function and your cognitive awareness.

You're probably wondering which foods will make you feel good—I'm sure you'd like a list of them so you can eat them every day! But the food-mood connection is different for everyone. A food such as oatmeal, which makes me feel great, may do nothing for you. And something like raisins, which leave me feeling tired and heavy, may be just the energetic pick-me-up that can fuel you through a long afternoon. So it's up to you to observe the effects of various foods on you and, through trial and error, to figure out what belongs on your plate. And remember that combinations count. Sometimes it's a combination of foods that affects you, so if you're feeling sluggish, look beyond individual foods.

To tease out the effects of various foods on your mood and attitude, keep a food-life inventory for about a week. Create a Food Assessment worksheet like the one on page 98 in your B.A.L.A.N.C.E. Journal. Write down all the foods you eat, along with the time you ate them, your moods throughout the day, your movement, and what's going on in your life.

Begin noticing how different types of foods make you feel. You'll probably discover that some foods make you feel good and others leave you sluggish and tired. That's important information for you to know as you create your own best balanced diet. One of my clients used to grab a candy bar at the grocery store when she'd stop after work to pick up food for dinner. Once she started paying attention, she noticed that having a candy bar on an empty stomach made her tired and cranky while she was making dinner. One day she skipped her pre-dinner candy bar and she realized she was less likely to snap at her kids while she cooked, although she was still starving. So she tried having a couple of peanut butter crackers instead of candy, and it made a huge difference in her mood. Once she realized all this, she found it easy to stop buying candy bars.

As you go along, scribble down any observations you may have about possible food-mood connections. If you notice that you feel great all morning when you have granola and fruit for breakfast but exhausted at ten A.M. when you breakfast on a bagel and jam, write it down. Then try both breakfasts again and see if the observations hold up. Continue to experiment with all the foods you commonly eat.

Make sure to hold on to this worksheet—we'll be referring back to it in Chapter 4.

Identifying Your Triggers

We all have trigger foods—treats like chocolate or cheese or salty chips—that we can't stop eating once we start. Say you're triggered by chocolate chip cookies. One small cookie may turn you into the cookie monster and create a binge that can last for weeks. For some people, certain foods can be addicting.

Use your Food Assessment Worksheet to help identify your trigger foods and decide whether there are foods you should avoid completely—

just as a recovering alcoholic has to stay away from liquor and a former smoker avoids cigarettes. Knowing your trigger foods and facing up to the power they hold over you will help you as you set out to balance your eating behaviors.

You probably also have trigger moments—out-of-balance situations that send you running for the refrigerator in an attempt to cope with stress, exhaustion, or worry. The Food Assessment Worksheet can also help you identify trigger moments and create plans to help you handle them in ways that will pave the way for you to feel calmer, lighter, and less likely to head for the kitchen.

Visualize Your Triggers

The act of imagining that you are eating a food you crave may help you eat less of it, according to a Carnegie Mellon study. Researchers found that people who visualized eating thirty bites of cheese, candy, and other high-crave foods ate 40 to 50 percent less of those foods than those who visualized eating just three bites.

What Are You Eating?

Being aware of what you are eating matters because you may discover that you are over- or under-fueling your body, taking in low-quality fuel, or fueling your body for reasons way deeper than physical hunger. Be sure to write down everything you eat, even the little bites—a handful here and a bite there can add up quickly. When you track your eating habits, you may notice that you're eating more than you realized.

Food Assessment Worksheet

Date	Meal	Food Eaten and Amount	Trigger Food (Yes or No)	Source of Food (super-market, fast-food place, restaurant)	Method of Preparation (packaged, made from scratch)	Mood Before and After Eating	Overall Outlook That Day	Observations About Food-Mood Connections

Assessment-Aiding Foods

In order to assess yourself, you must be in a calm, cool, collected sort of state. Assessing is about accepting who you are now, so as you work on this chapter, consider adding some nutrients that have soothing benefits to create calm in your life:

Make a soothing spread: Peel back an avocado and mash it up. Chop in some tomatoes, a sprinkle of sea salt and pepper, and then spread it on crackers, toast, or tortillas. The potassium in tomatoes and avocados will help soothe you.

Create a calming mix: Combine dark, leafy greens such as chard with chopped artichoke and chopped egg whites to create a salad mix full of calming B vitamins and magnesium. These nutrients help convert the amino acid tryptophan, which is found in egg whites, into serotonin, a brain chemical that helps your body calm down, unwind, and relax.

Take time for tea: L-theanine, a compound found in tea leaves, is thought to promote relaxation and enhance mood by stimulating the production of alpha brain waves. Tea (especially green tea) also contains compounds that may help reduce blood pressure, prevent hypertension, rev up metabolism, and promote weight loss.

Assessing Your Internal Muscle

Transformation absolutely begins within your heart and your mind. Your attitude, the way you process information, and your core values all create your internal muscle. Just like physical muscles, the internal muscle needs to be worked out, stretched, and practiced daily. Assess your internal muscle by taking the following steps:

1. **Core values:** Using your core values from Chapter 2, write a list of ways you currently honor each of them. For example, if a core value is giving and you tithe, note it here.

   Create a **Core Values Expression Assessment** that looks like this:

   Core Values Expression Assessment

Core Value	Expressed By . . .	Frequency?
Giving	Volunteering at the food pantry	1 × per week

2. **Internal strength:** List all the sources of internal strengthening that you currently partake in or have experienced within the last three months, along with the date or time frame. Also note if it has had a positive, negative, or neutral effect on you. Some examples are seeing a coach, counselor, therapist, or business advisor; reading self-development books; partaking in online or in-person communities focused on growth; and so forth. If you feel fulfillment, healing, support, or forward movement, the activity has a positive effect. If you feel confused, frustrated, empty, or angry, it probably has a negative effect on you. And if you simply don't know or you feel like it's a take-it-or-leave-it activity, call it a neutral. Also add any notes that come to mind while assessing these activities.

Here is an example from a client's B.A.L.A.N.C.E. Journal:

1. Read *The Shift* by Dr. Wayne Dyer (1 time) + loved the book, should reread it

2. Working out at Curves (3–4 times per week) + feel supported and strong

3. Meeting with support group (1 time per week) + they know me so well

4. Joined online social media group (3 times)—don't understand how it works

Anything you consider mental strengthening should go on this list. Hold on to it, because we will revisit it throughout the book.

B.A.L.A.N.C.E. Tip

Balance Doing and Being

Our life is made up of moments when we are either doing or being. Our human nature calls for us to balance both. The doing side of us is the force that drives us to make lists, set alarms, go to work, move our feet, and so on. The being side of us is the philosopher, the wonderer, and the romantic who likes to look at the night sky, cuddle on the couch, lie on the beach, and listen to music. Tilting too far toward either side—too much doing or too much being—puts us off balance. If you're spending so much time running errands and not enough time smelling the roses—or vice versa—try righting the doing/being balance by shifting your focus to a more centered approach. Make time each day to do and to be.

Assessing Should Be
a Judgment-Free Zone

Recently, I was meeting with Amanda to go over her Core Values Expression Assessment. When I arrived at our meeting, she looked a little ashamed as she showed me her blank chart. She said, "Jennifer, I tried to do this assessment, but it just made me sad. So many of the values excited me, but I know I'm not doing anything to express them."

I reminded Amanda of the two important rules about assessing:

1. Never judge yourself.

2. Don't try to "fix" anything.

Amanda smiled as she recalled these rules, and with this signal that it was okay to move forward, I asked Amanda which values excited her, and we decided to do the sheet together. She began with giving. She has a therapy dog, Deja, and she told me that she used to take her to local nursing homes. It's a value, and she's expressed it—I told her to write it down, along with the frequency. She also decided to acknowledge the date she last expressed the value, which was almost two years ago. Just by speaking about it, Amanda was excited to begin bringing Deja again!

Next, she chose creativity. Amanda had recently begun a crochet class with her mother, and she had been crocheting daily. She also liked to make jewelry and just recently made two bracelets. She also figured that because she loved to make jewelry and she valued giving, perhaps she could begin selling jewelry for a cause and donating a portion of her proceeds to an organization. Amanda's eyes lit up as she discussed the possibilities. While assessment is about no judgment or overthinking the *how*, if an idea pops into your head, go for it!

The value Amanda chose next was family. She said she expresses the family value by spending time with her parents and husband. I looked around her home and noticed photos everywhere of her family—displaying the photos was another expression of this value. Again, Amanda was exhilarated by her self-discovery that she was already expressing her values but just hadn't been acknowledging how.

When it came to friendship, she determined that she expressed the value by phone calls, e-mails, and monthly outings. While she had been pretty busy and she wished she had more time for her friendships, she did feel good that she kept strong relationships with her best friends. Yet another idea came out while we were chatting— Amanda figured she could express her creativity value and make more jewelry, which she could send to her friends during her busy times. She'd include a simple note that she's thinking of them and couldn't wait for their next get-together!

Assessing Your Schedule

Is a frantic schedule preventing you from living a balanced life? Are you so busy working, taking care of other people, and keeping up with all your personal and professional responsibilities that you don't have time to eat well, exercise, nurture yourself, spend time with friends and family, and enjoy your life?

Being crunched on time can often lead to being out of balance in life and on the scale. If you're so strapped for time that you feel you can't live the life you want, don't worry. You *can* take control of your schedule and find time for yourself. But in order to do this, you'll have to change the way you think about time.

I remember once thinking that time had to be managed and that this meant squeezing more tasks into less time—balancing your checkbook while gulping down dinner, loading the dishwasher while you talk to your mom on the phone, doing conference calls while you're driving your kids to soccer practice, or learning Spanish while running on the treadmill. But that's not a balanced approach, and it may even lead to less appreciation for life. Utilizing your time in a balanced way is not about learning how to juggle more, better, and faster.

Balancing your time means taking a good hard look at how you spend your time and making tough decisions about how you *really* want to use the minutes, hours, and days of your life. It's about asking for help and delegating responsibilities, learning to say no, saying yes with mindfulness, grouping tasks into efficient bundles, and rearranging your schedule according to your most important priorities. It means putting your life first and adding in tasks rather than trying to squeeze your life into the tiny bits of empty space in your calendar.

When you learn the true value of your time and make the choice of how you want to spend it, you'll feel calmer and less stressed, your life will open up, and the scale will go down. You'll find time for that art class you've wanted to take, that movie you've been dying to see, and the date you and your husband have been planning for the past two years. By taking control of your schedule, you'll give yourself the gift of time.

TAKE ACTION

. . . .

DO A DAY DUMP

The first step to balancing your time is becoming conscious of what you do every day. The Day Dump Worksheet is a great tool for this task.

Pour yourself a cup of coffee, tea, or water with lemon. (I don't suggest a glass of wine for this activity because you have to be on your toes to get the most out of it.) Gather up a pen and paper (or if you prefer, a computer with a spreadsheet program), all your scheduling tools (day planner, calendar, smart phone, online calendar, and so on), along with four markers (red, green, blue, and pink). Find a quiet space where you can concentrate.

On your paper or spreadsheet, create eight columns. Label them with the seven days of the week. Label the eighth column *miscellaneous*. Your page should look something like this:

Day Dump Worksheet

Monday	Tuesday	Wednesday	Thursday	Friday	Saturday	Sunday	Miscellaneous

Next, start writing. List everything you do every day of the week, from morning till night. Include even the most mundane tasks, such as brushing your teeth and tying your kids' shoes. Write it *all* down. The more specific you can be, the better, because little things can take much more time than you realize. You may want to take a look at the Balanced Inspirista graphic at the beginning of the chapter—the little outer circles are the lifestyle factors. When you're doing your day dump, remember to factor in everything you do in all areas of your life.

When you finish, take a look at your lists. You will probably be amazed to see how much you do every day and to see it all written down in black and white. No wonder you feel so exhausted—you're probably doing the work of two or three women! No wonder you don't have time to take good care of your body.

Now grab your colored markers. It's time to start paring down your daily task load. Ask yourself these four questions:

1. **Which of these tasks can I delegate?** Grab your pink marker and highlight the tasks that someone else can do. Are you making lunches while your teens are playing video games? Are you folding laundry while your boyfriend is catching up on ESPN? Are you and your neighbor both driving to the same ballet classes and baseball practices? Are you giving your kids rides to places they can get to by foot or bicycle? At work, are you doing jobs that could be done by coworkers? Are you making elaborate homemade dinners with friends when everyone would be just as happy with a potluck? Are you putting together the entire PTA bulletin board alone when other moms are able to help? I'm sure some mommies would love to contribute and cut out shapes while you staple the backdrop!

   Delegating can be hard. You have to ask for help from people who may not be all that willing to chip in. You have to accept that others may not do the job as well as you would—for example, if your husband puts away the laundry, you have to accept that he may not share your feelings about the best way to fold a towel. If your kids unload the dishwasher, they may not stack the pots and pans in size order the way you do. But that's okay. What matters is that *you have more time,* not that your kitchen cabinets are arranged with military precision.

It may also surprise you how willing people are to chip in on the responsibilities, and (this will really shock you) they may even *want* to do stuff. They may even do things better than you do! I know when I first got married, I quickly found out that my husband was very good at some household chores, even better than I was. He was so used to doing things for himself, he enjoyed doing laundry and cleaning. Come to find out, he is a far better towel folder than I am, and he cleans corners like nobody else can. He's a regular old domesticated dad, and he loves it! Now, why would I take that joy away from him?

2. **Which of these tasks can I group together?** With your blue marker, highlight the tasks that can be grouped together to save time. Are there some things that you can clump together? For example, if you are spending too much time cooking and preparing lunches every day, consider doing a few days' worth of prep work on Sunday nights. Chop veggies, cook chicken, or freeze some casseroles, stews, or soups. You get the idea. This will free up morning time and evening time. Or do your workouts on your lunch hour instead of taking time at night or skipping the gym entirely. When you drop your daughter off at dance class, go food shopping and fill the car with gas to save time on the weekend. Clumping can make life easier if you do it in a way that works for you.

   If you prefer to have a little free time every night, clump less to spread out activities more. If you prefer having a few hectic days in order to have chunks of free time on other days, clump more. Do what makes the most sense for you.

3. **Which of these tasks can I eliminate?** Using your red pen, cross out the tasks that you no longer have to do (or want to do). If

you're always the go-to gal for PTA event planning but are bored with baking for meeting nights, gracefully announce that you're no longer available for cupcake duty. If keeping your yard perfectly landscaped has become a chore, put away the clippers and let the yard look wild sometimes. If stopping for morning coffee adds fifteen minutes to your day, get out your Mr. Coffee and brew at home.

Eliminating can be even harder than delegating. It's so easy to look at a task and say, "I can't stop doing that!" But you can! I guarantee there are things on your daily to-do list that you can cut. Think about it. Do you really have to have *lengthy* conversations on the phone (especially when they are filled with gossip)?

4.   **What are my priorities?** Now, using your green pen, highlight the tasks that you can't eliminate, group, or delegate. These are the activities you have to do. If you're looking at the list and thinking, *This really isn't a priority*, find a way to eliminate, group, or delegate it.

We will use this activity in future sections, so sit tight and smile wide—we just assessed your time, and hopefully you have more of it already.

· ·

B.A.L.A.N.C.E. Tip

Dance, Dance, Dance

When I'm feeling crunched for time, I like to do something completely and totally silly. Sometimes I dance around the room singing a funny song completely off-key. It interrupts that feeling of being overwhelmed, and it reminds me to try to have fun despite the stress in my life. Plus, it gives me energy, gets my blood flowing, and stretches my muscles a bit. When you're feeling stressed, get up and dance!

✧ Success Story

One of our Curves members once complained about constantly having no time. When we did the Day Dump Worksheet, we could plainly
see why. Her daughter was involved in nine extracurricular activities.
Yes, nine! Every day, she chauffeured her daughter to ballet, softball,
piano practice, and who knows what else. She was also expected to
help out by volunteering, donating, and fund-raising. This woman was
not only exhausted but also nearly broke, with no time or money for
herself.

I suggested she cut back her daughter's activities. At first, she ar-
gued that she couldn't—to be competitive, she said, her daughter
had to be involved in all these things. She also said it would break her
daughter's heart to ask her to give up any activities. She felt that as a
good mother, she couldn't say no to her daughter.

I recommended that she sit down and have a talk with her daughter
about the amount of time, money, and sacrifice all these activities required. Much to her surprise, her daughter understood completely.
She was tired of running around, too, but she hadn't wanted to let
her mother down by quitting! Her daughter picked her favorite activities, crossed out the rest, and soon they both felt happier and more
balanced. They even had enough time and money to go out for an
occasional mother-daughter dinner and shopping night.

Everyday B.A.L.A.N.C.E. Technique:
Accept

Situations and circumstances in life are often beyond our control. We
make mistakes. We fall down. We will fail. We are human.

I often used to spin my mental wheels and reach for comfort food when I was confronted with a difficult situation—a disagreement with a friend, a failed relationship, an empty bank account.

I even spent a number of years focusing mainly on my physical flaws—my dress size, the shape of my nose, the curl in my hair. I couldn't accept myself, and that caused me to waste so much mental energy. When I realized this, I decided to try to do a better job of accepting myself just as I am. Accepting became part of my everyday balance mantra, and it is much healthier than beating myself up over my flaws.

Accepting Situations or Circumstances

"Serenity is not freedom from the storm, but peace within the storm." I love this Native American proverb; it has meant so much in my life. I have it posted on my refrigerator to serve as a way to keep me grounded during turbulent times.

In a class I was teaching, I asked the ladies to name their most common cause of stress. One woman responded, "Stress comes from other people. People cause me stress." She then went on to list the various distressing things people had done to her. All were valid and beyond her control. Other top stressors included finances, lack of time, and impossible expectations.

Stress is hard to define—the dictionary lists ten meanings for the word. But too often we let stress define us.

What can you do if you have a daughter who is bulimic, a father who is an addict, a friend who doesn't seem to care about you, or a boss who keeps piling work on? Do you disown your family and friends, quit your job, and move to the nearest bubble? Hmm . . . maybe you've felt like it, but it's obviously unrealistic, right?

We can often feel stressed even in less extreme scenarios. Try this one: your husband lost his job, you are two months late on your bills, your kids are in a million activities, and you have volunteered for one too many fund-raisers. You can't move to an island and seclude yourself from the realities of life. But there are some ways to find "peace within the storm," as the proverb suggests.

Learning to Be Still

Stillness quiets the mind and centers you in the present moment. Although it takes some practice, stillness can give you a mental break from everything flowing through your brain—past worries, future concerns, and daily to-do lists. To practice stillness, find a space to just be—sitting under a tree in your yard, kneeling by the window, perched on your front step, soaking in a warm tub— whatever feels peaceful to you. Practice stillness regularly as a means of accepting. And remember, stillness includes listening. We may not know the answers, but sometimes when we listen, we hear the next step.

Embracing Lessons

I've learned we have to detach ourselves from the problems and embrace them in the moment as an integral part of our lives. We usually think about the lesson after the problem has been resolved or enough time has passed for us to come to terms with it. Be open to the lesson. Show gratitude and always give yourself space for tears, venting, and acceptance. Be gentle with yourself and others.

Staying Connected

Detach from letting the situation define you and connect to the world around you. For example, if the economy is personally affecting you (as it is millions of Americans right now), you can still have fun with your family, dance around the room, watch a great movie, laugh, and say hi to a stranger. And if loved ones are struggling with something— illness, personal issues, a job loss—spend time with them, read together, reminisce, and create. Each moment carries perfection and imperfection—both are beautiful in their own right. Our circumstances should not stop us from loving life—it is a gift.

TAKE ACTION

PRACTICE SELF-ACCEPTANCE

Sit down with your B.A.L.A.N.C.E. Journal and spend a few minutes writing about your perceived flaws and what you are working on accepting—physical imperfections, personality traits, or circumstances. Do you accept them, or do you waste energy wishing you could change the unchangeable? What flaw would you most like to learn to accept?

Of course, there's a difference between self-acceptance and plain old giving up. Each of us has to define our own acceptance standards. Here is one of mine:

> *I accept that my hips are a bit wider since I had my children, but I won't use that as an excuse to feed my body junk. As long as I nurture, honor, and respect myself from the inside, meaning the way I fuel my body and the way I treat myself emotionally, the outside will take care of itself perfectly as it should.*

What are your acceptance standards?

My Acceptance Pledge to My Children

My daughter asked me if she could begin ballet classes. This made me recall an incident in a coffee shop years ago when I overheard some mothers talking about ballet photos in front of their daughters.

One mother warned the other, "Make sure you pay the extra ten dollars to airbrush your daughter's flyaway hair and skin. I did my daughter's last year, and they came out amazing."

I was surprised to hear this, although I know that women are hard on themselves. It's difficult not to be with the impossible standards women have to deal with in magazines, on TV, and in the countless number of ways we believe we must be more perfect. But overhearing this conversation made me realize that these standards are now trickling down to children at younger and younger ages.

So I started to think about the pressures my daughter will be introduced to, very soon. I've always known that it's my job to give her a good, solid foundation of confidence and self-love from the inside out. I love every bit of her, and so should she. Even with my Lu's wild mane of curly locks, flyaways galore, I couldn't imagine even wanting to airbrush them out. Honestly, aren't those the things we look back on with a smile?

I distinctly remember my first ballet photo. My hair was a bit of a mess and I didn't wear a drop of makeup. My mother was in the hospital, and she was the only one I would allow to do my makeup. "No Mommy, no makeup!" I said. I adored my mother, and I still do.

But loving our daughters is not enough. They have to see us love ourselves. Parenting happens best when we are being, not telling, doing, or saying. Experience is the greatest teacher. So if I am to stay true to setting a solid self-love foundation, I must always practice self-love. I must continue to be confident and strong. My daughter must not hear or see me pick myself apart, and in order to do that, I must simply not pick myself apart. I must love myself as I am.

This is my promise, my pledge to my daughter—and to my son too. Here are some of the things I must do to keep this pledge, which will teach them to love themselves and be the person they were each born to be.

I pledge to take care of myself. Moms need self-care too. This means eating well, moving our bodies, taking time for little indulgences (even as simple as a long, hot bath). I work with thousands of women, and most of them do everything for everyone else and find very little time to practice self-care. Our self-worth is molded from the day we are born, and so is the self-worth our children develop. Daughters soon become mothers. If we're constantly told we're not good enough the way we are, then we naturally begin to feel unworthy and we take less care of ourselves, which trickles to everyone else in our lives. Our children pick up this negativity. But if we feel fabulous, it helps everyone in the family feel fabulous. I will take care of myself so I can be the best mom and example to my children.

I pledge to put people above things. Success in my life means much more than a career or financial gains. Much of how I measure success is by love—how much I can give and receive. It's really all you need (as John Lennon said). But when we give *of* ourselves, we actually are giving *to* ourselves. We give ourselves a richness in spirit, a feeling of self-love and value. This leads to abundance in all areas of our lives. I want my children to be givers, to give to the world, to value our family and their friendships and strangers on the street. To teach them this, I will put people first above the material things. I will help others and lend a hand, an ear, spare change, or time. I will communicate. I will connect.

I pledge to love the flaws: mine, theirs, and everyone's. Home should be a safe place, where we can let our hair down, wash off our makeup, and just be ourselves, embraced for who we are as individuals. After all, our unique beauty is in our flaws—inside and out. I must love mine, I must love my children's, and I must love everyone's. If Lu or the Man see me being harsh on myself or others, they will in turn look at themselves harshly.

I pledge to live with passion, purpose, and intention. When we live with passion, purpose, and intention, then confidence just sits comfortably in our hearts. There is no trying to be confident. We just are. I have a purpose here on this earth. We all do. Sometimes we can get bogged down in the burden of finding our purpose, but I think it unfolds naturally when we live with passion. Purpose may evolve and change, and even if we don't know our purpose fully, we can be passionate about life and all its twists and turns. I

will live with passion, believe in my purpose, and live with intention. Teaching this to my children is in and of itself one of the
greatest gifts I can give them, as my parents gave to me.

I pledge to be a visionary and to follow through. When we have
dreams, visions for our life that we put into motion, our confidence
comes naturally from within. I know that many times, mothers
and fathers put their dreams on hold to be caretakers. But I believe we must still have dreams and visions. I'm not talking about
haphazardly chasing a crazy dream. I'm talking about using our
natural talents, our unique gifts.

So, for me, this means I must take inspired actions and risks,
be fearless, and believe in my power. I must have faith. I must
pray and meditate—speak to God and listen. This will teach my
children that they can dream and achieve anything they want.
Even when we reach small goals, we create small changes, and
we enjoy a boost in confidence when we achieve bigger goals and
create bigger changes.

I pledge to learn and to try again when I fail. Failure can be
discouraging if we let it stop us, but it is necessary on the path of
self-growth and teaching children self-love. Whenever we fail, we
have an amazing opportunity to learn and grow. When we believe
in ourselves enough to try again, self-love manifests without question. I will teach my children that they can fly. But like a baby
bird, they will fall a bunch of times, maybe even break a wing.
Then eventually—with practice as well as failure, mistakes to
learn from, and tenacity—they will soar.

Summing Up

In this chapter, we've discussed the benefits of using self-assessment
of your body, your mind, your self-care, and your schedule in order to

find areas in your life that lack balance. I also suggested some strategies for self-acceptance. The activities I suggested included:

- Do a full assessment of your body and your health.

- Call your doctor and schedule a full physical.

- Assess your eating habits by keeping track of everything you eat for about a week.

- Do a day dump to help you clean out your schedule by pinpointing tasks that can be delegated, clumped, or eliminated.

- Create your acceptance standards and write an acceptance pledge to yourself or your loved ones.

In Chapter 4, I'll guide you through a process of letting go of more unnecessary baggage, and I'll tell you how learning to say one tiny word can instantly add balance to your life.

· ·

Chapter Four

L is for
Let Go and *Laugh*

Some people believe holding on and hanging in there are
signs of great strength. However, there are times when it takes
much more strength to know when to let go—and then do it.

—Ann Landers

· ·

M
y husband loves to garden, so he knows that before he can
plant anything, he's got to clear the ground—pull weeds,
remove rocks, yank old roots, and rake away dead leaves
and broken branches. Before new plants can grow, he's got to rid the
garden of all the debris that might prevent vulnerable young seedlings
from receiving the sunlight and rain they need to survive and thrive.

That's exactly what has to happen when you set out to rebalance
your life and your diet. Before you start making life-changing shifts
and building exciting new habits, you've got to clear away physical and
emotional debris so that as you plant the seeds of change, they have
the space they need to grow.

I refer to this as a cleansing process because it is an opportunity to let go or get rid of some of the foods, thoughts, and behaviors that can be toxic to you as you follow the B.A.L.A.N.C.E. Program.

Letting go can feel liberating and exciting. It's a chance to eliminate what's no longer serving a purpose, what's simply not serving you well, or what doesn't align with your core values and to start fresh. It's a technique you can use throughout your life, but it's especially important now, as you set out on your balance journey.

Let Go to Let In

The letting-go process is a comprehensive food-life cleanse that will help you release the foods, habits, and out-of-balance life choices that have weighed you down for so long. It also signifies your commitment to yourself and to your personal transformation. It's very powerful to choose what you want to let go in order to become who you were born to be.

As you get started, be sure you have your B.A.L.A.N.C.E. Journal by your side. Some of the activities you've done in previous chapters will help you determine what you need to let go of.

One important caveat before we start paring down: it's best to go through this process in a way that feels comfortable to you. The idea of a wholesale clearance is very scary to some people, and that's okay. If you're not the love-to-let-go type, start by simply reading this chapter, mulling over the recommendations, and applying them to you when and how you think would be best for you. But do keep in mind that the reason to go through a process of letting go is so you can make room to add important things that bring balance to your eating habits and your life. After we finish letting go in this chapter, we'll begin adding in the next chapter.

You'll be surprised how light and free you'll feel once you start letting go.

I remember when I chose to really cleanse my body for the first time—not because a diet prescribed a specific cleanse and not because

I was trying to lose weight, but because I felt an internal need to cleanse myself, because I wanted to nurture my body in a way I hadn't in such a long time. In my mind, the cleanse would last one week. It wasn't totally extreme; I just wanted to rid my body of processed foods. I decided to eat only whole foods—nothing from a package or with a list of ingredients. I had to know what was in everything I ate and be able to identify its source.

It made me feel so incredible! My energy soared, and I felt so good that it basically became my new way of living. And that was over a decade ago. The funniest thing was, I had no expectation of that. The cleanse just felt right for my body. And then the cleansing expanded into all other areas of my life, even my thought processes as I let go of self-limiting beliefs. It was exhilarating.

As I began working with clients, I realized that many of them were holding on to behaviors that no longer served their life vision. In my personal life as well, I learned the importance of letting go in many ways—whether it came to food choices, relationships, thoughts, or even material possessions. Letting go is a powerful tool to make space for what's yet to come, and it became an integral part of the B.A.L.A.N.C.E. Program.

In this chapter, I'll guide you through a series of letting-go steps.

First we'll do a **food cleanse** to help you rid your diet of foods that simply do not serve a greater purpose: healthy fuel, mood, energy, tradition, or simple pleasure. We will also do some simple switches and begin to eliminate trigger foods. Next we'll go through a thorough **cabinet and closet cutback** in your home, clearing out the excess junk to determine what to donate, shred, repurpose, recycle, sell, or toss in the trash. Then we will figure out how to **eliminate your time vacuums** to help you let go of some of the things that unnecessarily suck time out of your life. Finally we'll do a **mind-set purification** to let go of self-limiting beliefs and unhealthy thoughts that are holding you back from being in balance.

At the end of the chapter, you'll learn about the Everyday B.A.L.A.N.C.E. Technique, **laugh,** and why it really is the best medicine.

⚙ You've Been Lied To!

I constantly hear from women who are frustrated by the scale. I'm not a weight person. As a matter of fact, I say throw the darn scale away! According to Lindsay Vastola, certified fitness trainer and founder of Body Project Fitness & Health, not only is the scale an enemy to many women, it's also a liar. "And," Lindsay says, "we trust it enough to get naked for it. . . ."

Here are the lies that Lindsay warns us to watch out for:

1. **Weight loss always equals fat loss.** When you drop weight after a week of dieting or severe calorie restriction, the scale doesn't tell you that you've mostly shed excess water weight and precious muscle, *not* necessarily body fat. Bummer. This is why yo-yo dieting never, never, never works and why you are frustrated, frustrated, frustrated because you can't seem to maintain a healthy weight range.

2. **You can believe the scale.** The scale fails to tell you what the number it gives actually means. Your body composition is simply what makes up your total body weight, including water, body fat, muscle, organs and tissues, and your skeletal system. When you weigh on a standard scale, the number includes the total weight of all these components. This number can fluctuate for several reasons, often up or down by five pounds each day. It can change depending on hormonal levels during the month (especially for women); increased or decreased muscle mass (ladies, listen up: you may weigh more but look leaner when you have more muscle); changes in body fat, water retention, or temperature; transition in habits; or lack of sleep (which can lead to overeating).

3. **Good numbers equal good health.** Your weight does not give you a complete picture of how good you feel or how

healthy you actually are inside. Don't get me wrong—we shouldn't completely discount our total weight. It can be used as a baseline to our overall health. But if you're remaining consistent with a fitness routine and a well-balanced eating routine (even living it up a little), your focus seems to shift from the scale to how you're looking and feeling. I can almost guarantee if you asked ten fitness trainers or athletes if they ever weigh themselves, I bet eight out of ten say they don't. Why? Because they listen to their bodies—they are in tune with them enough to know when they're lacking energy or consuming too much or too little. They don't need a scale to tell them this.

Let go of using the scale as the only measurement of your success. Focus on how you feel in your clothes and how you evaluate your energy, your sleep, your mood, and your confidence. Avoid weighing daily—weigh once a week at most. You will know if you have gained weight when you look in the mirror or if those pants feel a little tighter than they did last winter. You will also know your body composition has changed if those pants feel a bit looser.

Free yourself from being a slave to the scale. It may not be an easy habit to break at first, but it will be the most liberating feeling when you finally do.

Your Food Cleanse

We're used to eating for the scale, thinking of foods as either good or bad based on how they impact our weight rather than how they nourish our bodies and impacts our lives.

Going through a food cleanse helps bring you back to a place in which you really connect to the fuel aspect of food. When you think of food only as an emotional tool, it's easy to lose track of the biological connection between food and your body. As you go through a multi-level food cleanse, the emphasis can start to shift back to food's most important function: keeping you alive and thriving.

Cleansing allows your taste buds to take a break from all the processed, over-salted, super-sugary foods we mindlessly eat and become reacquainted with the naturally delicious flavor of simple, nutritious foods. Let go of eating salty, greasy fast food for a few days and you'll rediscover the delicious flavor of a piece of grilled fish flavored with a dribble of olive oil and some fresh herbs. Avoid the candy dish for a while and your taste buds will luxuriate in the tangy sweetness of a fresh raspberry.

During your food cleanse, you will mindfully eat as cleanly as you are able. You'll eliminate foods that bring nothing to your table, so to speak, and begin to choose foods that will enhance your mood, nourish your body, and cleanse you from the sugary, processed foods that are commonplace in society today.

After you've gotten back to basics with your foods, I'll show you how to tap in to your creative side and craft simple, beautiful, healthy, delicious meals that you can feel good about for the rest of your life.

How to Do a Personal Food Cleanse

Where you begin your food cleanse depends on where you are right now and how much you commit to cleansing your body. While a true food detoxification can take a number of different routes (some say eating only raw foods is a true cleanse, others say juicing, while others will tell you to eliminate carbohydrates, animal proteins, or dairy), the idea here is to release some of the pressure and simply begin where you feel comfortable.

Whenever possible, focus on eating natural, whole foods. Realize that food in its natural state is designed almost perfectly for digestion and is nutrient rich. For example, choose plain yogurt (I prefer Greek or coconut milk yogurt) over the flavored kind, even the fruit flavors. Connect with the creamy, natural texture. In many cases, flavored yogurt has two to three times more sugar.

I know what you're thinking: *plain yogurt—yuck!* I used to think that too. But your palate changes when you begin eating food in a more natural state. I used to be *in love* with yogurt that had highly sweetened fruit already mixed in, and I despised the taste of plain yogurt. Now I am quite the opposite. I don't enjoy sugary yogurts and can't stomach the taste of artificially sweetened ones. Plain yogurt is a blank canvas—you can use your creativity to make it wonderful (and super-nutritious) with natural flavors and textures. If you love fruit, add in a half cup of blueberries, a pinch of stevia, and a dash of pure vanilla extract. When you're feeling tropical, add pure coconut extract and sliced strawberries. For the taste of decadence, add a bit of dark baker's cocoa, a pinch of stevia, a sprinkle of cinnamon, and a teaspoon of pure almond butter. If you love the taste of fruit-on-the-bottom yogurt, reduce frozen blueberries (or whatever fruit you fancy) on the stove, add some whole blueberries for texture, and top with plain yogurt mixed with pure vanilla extract. You'll never want to eat the other stuff again.

Cleanse your palate to enjoy food without processed sugars or artificial sweeteners. It's incredible when you realize that raw sugar is actually not that sweet. Refined white sugar is a bit sweeter, and the artificial varieties carry ten to twelve times the amount of sweetness and can often simulate a blood sugar response—not to mention all the other adverse effects! Too much sugar can contribute to tooth decay, cavities, and type 2 diabetes. Problems such as osteoporosis as well as vitamin and mineral deficiencies can also

Be Safe and Always Check

Be sure to check with your health care provider before embarking on a food cleanse, especially if you have diabetes, disordered eating, kidney disease, or any other chronic health condition. Pregnant women should follow their prenatal care provider's recommendations regarding diet and weight.

occur when your diet includes high-sugar foods instead of more nutritionally balanced foods. When you cleanse your body, you notice the sugar cravings often go away. I can't tell you how many clients are astonished at how drastically their cravings change—in a positive, healthy way.

To design a personal food cleanse that will be best for your body, consider eliminating the following foods:

4. **Moody foods.** Refer to the Food Assessment Worksheet from Chapter 3 and eliminate the foods that negatively affect your mood.

5. **Processed foods.** Use your Food Assessment Worksheet to think about how much processed food you eat. If it's a big part of your diet, cleanse out as much of it as possible this week. Choose real food over fake food. If you're eating highly processed white bread, switch to whole-grain bread. If you already eat pretty well, replace some refined grains with whole grains, switch instant flavored oatmeal for slow-cooked plain oats (sprinkle in some cinnamon and cut-up apples, and it's so delicious!). Here's a simple rule to remember—if it's instant, it's processed. If it cooks more quickly, the oat or grain has been stripped of the nutrients that come from the husk. Anything you do to begin cleansing your daily food intake will help move you in the right direction.

6. **Fast food.** Once again, check your Food Assessment Worksheet to help you evaluate how prevalent fast food is in your diet. If you find you have a soft spot for cheeseburgers and fries, make it a goal to let go of fast food this week. Don't go to extremes. If you practically live at the drive-through, cutting out a few fast food meals is a great beginning. If you always eat fries or chips as a side, order apple slices instead.

7. **Junk food.** The phrase *junk food* means different things to different people—to some it's potato chips and cupcakes, and to others it's anything that doesn't come from Whole Foods. Whatever your definition, try letting it go this week. Remember, this isn't about absolutes—you don't have to stop eating Ruffles forever. The beauty of the B.A.L.A.N.C.E. Program eating plan is that you can eat the foods you love. But just for this week, try leaving them and other junk food out of your diet during your food cleanse. In the next chapter, I'll suggest ways to add them back to your diet in a healthier, more balanced way as well as ways to create recipes with similar flavors and textures.

8. **Trigger foods.** The only foods I recommend you avoid completely are your trigger foods, those that trigger uncontrollable eating. Check your Food Assessment Worksheet for a list of your trigger foods. I'm not saying you can't ever have your trigger foods again. But taking them out of your diet (and your house) for a week helps enormously in the food cleanse process because it pushes you to honestly confront the way these foods impact your life.

B.A.L.A.N.C.E. Tip

Be Prepared

Create a shopping list before you leave the house so you can be prepared when you hit the food store or farmers market. You will save yourself time, money, and frustration. Being clear and focused will help you to choose foods that serve your body and life well.

Toxin-Cleansing Leafy Greens and Herb Mix

Apple cider vinegar, pine nuts, and herb blends have traditionally been used for detoxification. They are believed to help eliminate toxins, reduce the risk of disease, and assist in weight loss. You may be surprised to learn that many of your favorite foods also assist the body's detoxification systems, including the liver, intestines, kidneys, and skin. You can actually help ward off the harmful effects of pollution, food additives, secondhand smoke, and other toxins with a variety of delicious fruits, vegetables, nuts, oils, and beans. Here's a quick mix that is simple, healthy, and delicious:

Serves 1

What You'll Need

    2 tablespoons olive oil

    ¼ cup pine nuts

    1 cup dark leafy greens

    ½ cup herb blend

    2 tablespoons apple cider vinegar

    ½ teaspoon blackstrap molasses, or raw honey or sugar

Let's Do This

Start by toasting the pine nuts. In a small pan, drizzle 1 tablespoon of the olive oil and heat on medium high. Add the pine nuts and brown for 1½ to 2 minutes. Remove to a small bowl to cool, and set aside.

In a large salad bowl, toss together the dark, leafy greens and the herb blend.

In a separate small bowl, mix the apple cider vinegar with the remaining tablespoon olive oil and the blackstrap molasses. Whisk it together and then toss the dressing into your salad mix. Add the toasted pine nuts, sprinkle in some raisins, and you are in autumn salad heaven.

Options Galore

This combination of herbs, leafy greens, and apple cider vinaigrette is a light, simple, healthy, delicious meal. But it can also serve as a base that you can do so much with! If you want a protein boost, you can add white beans, grilled chicken, or even a little pancetta. If you want a creamy texture to balance the crisp herb blend, try adding goat cheese or warmed brie. If your sweet tooth is kicking in, add sliced apples and a hint of cinnamon. Use your imagination or just whatever is left in your refrigerator. Slice up some bananas or grapes, add provolone, chop up some more veggies, bake cinnamon-coated walnuts . . . there is no wrong way to make this salad. Be creative and enjoy!

Bonus Benefits

Leafy Greens and Herb Mix: Extremely low in calories but packed with nutritional benefits, leafy greens make a filling snack or meal and also cleanse the body. They are low in fat, high in fiber, and rich in folic acid, vitamin C, potassium, and magnesium. Leafy greens also contain many phytochemicals, such as lutein, beta-cryptoxanthin, zeaxanthin, and beta-carotene. Also containing antioxidants, dark, leafy greens have cancer-fighting properties.

Now that you've determined what foods to let go during your food cleanse, you're probably thinking what the heck you *can* eat this week. That's up to you, but I find that a great place to start is the perimeter of your grocery store. Shop around the outer edges, where the fresh fruits, vegetables, meats, and breads are, and then go from there! I also find it helps to ask yourself these three simple questions about each of your food choices:

1. Does this food choice **fuel** my body with healthy, pure ingredients loaded with nutrients?

2. Does this food choice elevate my **mood** before, during, and after I eat it?

3. Does this food choice boost and sustain my **energy** level?

If the answer to these questions is yes, the food you're considering is probably a good choice for your food cleanse week.

TAKE ACTION

READ THE FINE PRINT

When I started trying to balance my diet, I realized I knew very little about the food I was eating. I had been on so many diets for so long that I no longer thought about the nutrients in food—it was all about calories. In my mind, a low-calorie food was good, and a high-calorie food was bad. My eyes went straight to the calorie count on every food label.

That kind of thinking is completely out of balance, of course. I learned about nutrition and how the body works. Nutritious food positively impacts you in so many ways. Your mind and body need proteins, fats, carbohydrates, and a range of vitamins, minerals, antioxidants, and phytochemicals. Eating well is about a lot more than just how many calories a food has.

To reconnect with what's whole and healthy about food, start reading labels. Skip the calorie count and focus instead on a food's ingredients. If it's full of stuff you've never heard of, do some research and find out what those ingredients are and where they come from. Milk is from cows and eggs are from chickens, but what about things like maltodextrin? Get on the Internet and find out. (I'll let you off the hook on this one—maltodextrin is a food additive made through the hydrolysis of starch and is absorbed by your

What's on Your Table?

A recent Harvard study found that people who eat yogurt, nuts, fruits, and whole grains gain less weight over time than those who regularly eat potatoes, French fries, and white bread. Simple switches of what's on your table will do the trick.

body as rapidly as glucose is. So as far as your body is concerned, malto-dextrin is another word for sugar. But it is a processed sugar.)

I'm not saying you can't eat foods with unpronounceable names. But I do want you to think before you eat them. Understand what's in them, and then make a choice. You owe it to your body to be aware of what you're putting in it.

The Cabinet/Closet Cutback

While you cleanse your diet during the letting go step of the B.A.L.A.N.C.E. Program, it's also important to cleanse and detoxify your home. This doesn't mean throwing out the toxic cleaning supplies you keep under your sink—although that's not a bad idea. It means getting rid of the unnecessary, expired, or junk food in your refrigerator and cabinets and cutting back on the clutter in your closets.

Go through your cabinets and refrigerator and determine what food to clear out. Immediately place it in bags or boxes to donate or throw away. It's up to you to define the meaning of the phrase *junk food* for yourself because it varies tremendously, and again, its meaning depends on where you are in terms of your current diet. But let's be honest, you know it when you see it.

Again, I'm not saying you can never have this food again, although I find that many women I work with cleanse their taste buds and no longer want the stuff they once loved! But for now, clearing the junk food out of your house is a valuable step in the process of redefining your relationship with food. If it absolutely irks you to throw it out or give it away, then box it up and store it in the garage. You can figure out ways to use it later.

When one of my clients cleansed her body of processed pasta for a week, she didn't want to toss it because she figured she'd use it again. During that week she gave fresh pasta a try, and she loved it so much she never looked back! So what did she do with all that unused pasta in her garage? She gave it to her kids for crafting projects. They glued it onto inexpensive picture frames, painted and decorated them, and gave them to friends and family for gifts.

And of course, you can always donate nonperishable foods to a food pantry.

Family Matters

If you have a family, don't upset the entire household by cleansing out their favorite foods. Instead of removing everything, try creating a cabinet section with the foods you would be cleansing. I know that having foods in the house is a huge temptation, especially if "stress-eating" has become somewhat robotic for you. I've learned that even a moment of hesitation or thought, though, can stop stress-eating in its tracks. So, if you are visual, you may want to remind yourself in some sort of visual way that certain cabinet sections contain food options that you are choosing to cleanse from your body. You can put a picture of a cartoon character to remind you this food is for your children or a photo of a football to remind you the food is hubby's halftime snacks. If words work better for you, make a sign with the name(s) of the family member(s), or if you're a "quotes" person like me, write down an inspiring quote to remind you of your goals. Having a reminder system is very helpful to redirect you if and when you open the cabinet! I understand you may want everyone in your family to let go of junk food, but please remember that preaching healthy doesn't work—it simply makes people want to revolt. You can inspire others in your household to be healthy by modeling healthy behavior. When they see your increased energy, your more joyful demeanor, your overall lightness, trust me—they will want you to help them make some changes too.

Spring Cleaning Whatever the Season

Next, tackle the rest of your home with a thorough cleaning session. Dust the furniture, wash the windows, clean the bathrooms—I'm talking spring cleaning even if you're reading this in the dead of winter. Cleaning your home from top to bottom is a kind of renewal—it allows you to start fresh. When you're scrubbing the toilet, you're making a real commitment to your life change. It's kind of like flossing after you brush your teeth—you're less likely to have a snack because your teeth are clean. Cleaning out your home is a concrete, physical way to begin to clean out your life.

If that sounds overwhelming, take baby steps. Begin with one section of your home, one room, even just one drawer. Even if you start small, the feeling you get from cleansing your home will extend into other parts of your life. Denise began by just cleaning and polishing her silverware—just the knives, in fact. She felt good about it and liked the way they looked, so she moved on to the forks. Little by little, she cleansed her entire house, shed, and garage and is now working on her mother's house.

Redesign Your Life

Removing clutter can help you think more clearly: a Princeton University study recently found that visual clutter reduces your ability to focus and process information. Calmer energy, a sense of presence and balance, and sharper life focus can flourish in a decluttered home. Here are some simple ways to start cleansing clutter:

Set the stage. Go through your surroundings and take inventory. Is there a room that you aren't crazy about? Does it have wallpaper from the 1970s? A lightbulb that's not bright enough—or maybe a bit too bright? A hole in the wall? A squeaky door?

It doesn't cost much to put on a fresh coat of paint, fill holes, fix squeaks, and replace bulbs and batteries for a clean, updated look. And yet, it will make you feel so much better. And if design isn't your thing, flip through a magazine to find a picture of a room you love. Recreate the look yourself, and you'll save tons.

Choose colors carefully. Keep in mind that colors affect us more than we think. Pick colors that are conducive to what you want your space to be. If you want a serene room, stay away from red! Red is an energizer and may even stimulate your appetite. Greens are calming colors, perfect for a spa-inspired setting. Or if you want a cross between calm and amped up, choose a shade of blue.

Tackle your to-do list. We all have mental to-do lists, but now's the time to put it on paper and check it off. Make a list of the tasks that have been on your mind, like organizing a closet, filing cabinet, or drawer. Tackle the items one by one. Clearing clutter clears your mind too.

Store no more. Our closets, garages, and basements are havens for hidden treasures we may have written off too soon. You can go green and save green by refurbishing old furniture (it's amazing what furniture treatment and new hardware can do) or using bottles as decorative details (glass is said to be relaxing just to look through) to add a fresh new decor to your home. Be creative and you can design a whole new space with items you already own. Then cleanse your home and storage areas of what's not in use and no longer serves a purpose in your life.

Organize to organize. If you're trying to be organized, it may be overwhelming at first. Start simply by getting four bins and labeling them: *Use, Donate, Toss,* and *Shred.*

- Items in the *Use* bin should be put to use now!

- Donate items you no longer use by picking an organization of your choice. Many even offer free pickup services. Remember to clean them before donating!

- Toss whatever can't be used—either into the trash can or the recycling bin.

- Shred paperwork with private information and recycle it.

Eliminating Your Time Vacuums

In Chapter 3, you used the Day Dump Worksheet to delegate and eliminate time-consuming activities from your schedule. But you may still be finding that you have less time than you'd like.

We've all had days that were perfectly planned out but, for some reason, nothing—I mean nothing—on our to-do lists gets done. If you're finding that every day is feeling like it's getting sucked away by unplanned tasks, you're probably getting stuck in a time vacuum. Eliminating time vacuums will free up space for healthier habits, such as dance class, trips to Curves, nature hikes, home cooking, healthy baking, or even at-home spa treatments. It will also lower the levels of stress hormones in your body.

Take a lesson from Mariana. She didn't even come to me for weight issues. She simply wanted to regain a sense of balance in her life and her business. After about three months, she lost fifteen pounds without even trying very hard. She said she felt the weight melt off of her body as her stress levels came down. Mariana learned, as so many of my ladies do, that balance equals less stress, and less stress equals weight loss (even when weight loss isn't your number one goal).

So first check out your Day Dump Worksheet from Chapter 3 and see what you are delegating and/or taking off of your to-do list. Hold yourself accountable to implement what you determined and have the conversations necessary to delegate.

Here are some other common time vacuums. Are they sucking away your time?

1. **E-mail.** E-mail is one of the worst time vacuums ever. Items just keep popping up in your inbox, demanding immediate attention. But you can take control by putting a few rules into place.

    *   Create a folder system within your inbox for messages awaiting a reply. Prioritize the categories and calculate a reasonable response time.

    *   Create standard replies to inform senders that they may be waiting to hear from you and include the expected wait time.

    *   Delegate items when appropriate and delete junk or unsolicited nonessential items immediately. Don't waste time by checking out the latest dancing cat video, no matter how hilarious your friend promises it to be.

    *   If you're using e-mail for personal messages or fun, you may want to designate a time of day for e-mails.

    *   If you're anxiously awaiting something, you can use your phone to create an e-mail alert system so you don't always have to log in to the computer to find out if you've received the anticipated message.

2. **Surfing the web.** The Internet has revolutionized the way we do business, find information, connect with friends, share pictures, and even shop. But sometimes you get so sucked in, you can't get out. To avoid wasting time on the web, view the Internet as you would any other browsing activity. You wouldn't waste the day strolling around the mall when you are supposed to be at work. The same goes with the Internet.

If staying off-line is particularly difficult for you, log on only during specific browsing times. Set a time limit and use an alarm to remind you when your time is up.

3. **Talking on the phone.** Who doesn't love a good girlfriend heart-to-heart? I know I do! But if you have a lot of friends and they call you often, those calls can suck up hours a day. I know—I've filled many days with long phone calls. But if the phone is interfering with your fulfillment, or your chatter is on a negative path, perhaps it's time to hang up.

Phone calls were a big problem for Amy. She was super-motivated to lose weight. Every week she'd leave our meetings energized and excited. But she'd return the following week looking as if the dog ate her homework. Finally she admitted that every day after her kids left for school, she looked at her calendar, set her intentions, started moving . . . and then the phone would ring . . . and ring . . . and ring as one friend after another called. Most of the time the conversations amounted to little more than good-natured gossip—fun, but a time waster for my client, who was anxious to balance her life.

When Amy started letting those morning calls go to voice-mail, she had a lot more time to focus on her priorities: going to the gym, shopping at the farmers market, and making healthier meals. To be sure she stayed connected with her friends, she started a tradition of Sunday night potluck suppers that gave everyone plenty of time to chat.

Learning to Say No

You may have to let go of some things on your to-do list. There's one thing standing between you and balancing your time: the word *no*.

If you feel like there just aren't enough hours in the day to do everything on your list, it's most likely because you say yes to too many

Hearing the Word *No*

My mother is notorious for being a yes-woman. She wants to help everybody all the time with everything, and she often puts herself to last on the list. I have to admit that when I was younger, I loved that my mother would drop everything to help people—especially me—but as I got older (and wiser, of course) I began to see that my mother was overextending herself. And I noticed I was doing it too! I was saying yes to everyone, and when I said no, I would spend days or weeks agonizing, feeling guilty, and apologizing.

I realized Mom and I were caught in an exhausting cycle: the Yes-No-Guilt-Exhaustion Cycle. I asked too much of her. She had trouble saying no to me, and when she did, I felt disappointed. This made her feel guilty. We had to stop this—I had to learn to ask for less, she had to get better at saying no, and we both needed to stop feeling guilty.

Now, I remind her it's okay to say no when I ask her to watch my kids or support me in some other way. It's a good reminder that I have to say no more often too. Being aware, conscious, and considerate of her boundaries has opened me up to being more conscious of my own—and that's benefitted both of us.

things and, as a result, you're overextended. There's no way to jam more hours in a day. The only way to free up time to take care of yourself is to stop doing something—and the way to do that is to say no more often. Imagine yourself being pulled and stretched until you are almost unrecognizable—even elastic loses its "snap" at some point. Saying no will bring your life back into proportion.

Saying no is one of the most powerful ways to balance your schedule and your life. But *no* can also be one of the hardest words to say. It can make you feel selfish, negative, self-centered, uncaring, and guilty. But if you're saying no to avoid dumping time into something you don't have time for, you're not being selfish. You're making an investment in a better life.

The best way to say no is to combine it with a reason or an alternate solution. If you can't think of a way to say no, give yourself time by saying maybe. Here's an example: Your neighbor asks you to take care of her dog for a week while she's on vacation. This would involve feeding the dog and walking him two or three times a day. Here are three ways to say no:

- No, because my new job is keeping me so busy, I simply don't have the time to take proper care of Fido.

- No, but I bet that teenager down the street would be happy to earn a few bucks taking care of your dog.

- I'll call you later and let you know—I have to check my schedule.

Resist the urge to lie when you want to say no. And don't apologize—you have a right to choose what you do and don't have time for.

Saying no isn't limited to requests by other people. You may have to say no to yourself too. Taking care of your neighbor's pup may appeal to you—perhaps you're a dog lover living in an apartment with a no-pets policy. But your schedule is already so full that adding another task would put you over the edge. Say no, but offer to take the dog for a long walk some Saturday morning when you have plenty of time. Or say no to something else in your schedule to add in some time for pure joy with the puppy.

TAKE ACTION

CONNECT WITHOUT JUDGMENT

Many women are incredibly self-judgmental. We criticize ourselves, obsess over even the smallest of flaws, blame ourselves for things that aren't even our fault, and beat ourselves up over the smallest mistakes. If we spoke to other people that way, they would feel awful!

Learning not to judge ourselves is a complicated process that we'll discuss throughout the book. But right now, a very simple and fulfilling way to start tackling all that negative self-judgment is to do an activity I call connecting without judgment.

Here's how it works: For the next week, give something wonderful to everyone you come across. Everyone—your spouse, your kids, your neighbors, the people at work, the bus driver, the guy who cleans your office, the cop directing traffic, the dry cleaner—you get the idea. Give them all a gift: a smile, a positive vibe, a quick silent prayer, a hug, a pat on the back, or a word of encouragement. It doesn't matter what it is as long as it's something positive.

By doing this, you start to accept, in a very small way, that everyone deserves the gift of love without judgment. When you're smiling at someone, you're less likely to judge them. You're nurturing them without judgment. If you can learn how to do this with others, it will become easier for you to do it for yourself.

· ·

Mind-Set Purification

Our mind-set has a very powerful effect over our being. One of my favorite writers, philosophers, and teachers, Douglas Pittman, says, in his book *Principles for Living on the Edge,* "It is estimated that half of the content of our mind, the beliefs, the judgments, and the programs that operate our autopilot are in place by the time we are four years old . . . by the time we are eight years old as much as 80 percent of our belief systems are in place. . . . And as much as 95 percent of our daily actions are generated from this content of our mind, albeit unconsciously."

We all have ingrained thoughts and beliefs about life, health, wellness, nutritious eating, and weight. Many are simply self-limiting beliefs. These self-limiting beliefs can easily turn into excuses that block us from finding balance and good health.

I always used to say I was just big boned and that my body couldn't lose weight because of the way I was built. I don't know why I thought that, but I truly believed it. When my body changed and my weight went down, I proved myself wrong. I nurtured myself, and my body responded. And I realized my bones are my bones—I'm not sure if they are big or small, but it doesn't matter anyway!

It's important to recognize our beliefs and then to test them to determine whether they're true or false. If they're true based on an indisputable fact and they are working for you in your life, stick with them. But if your beliefs are false or they have become roadblocks, you'll need to let them go and educate yourself so you can replace them with a true, effective set of beliefs. Clinging to a belief system based on failure makes success impossible.

Once I met a woman named Nina. She told me she could never work out. I asked her why and she said she was too arthritic and she would damage her body more. She said working out was too painful and she was too old to take on the burden anyway. The more I tried to tell her working out would help her, the more she resisted my advice. "It's not an excuse, Jennifer! It's true. I can't do it." Rather than arguing the point, I encouraged her to just open her mind, to educate herself about arthritis and natural ways to relieve the pain, and to let me know what she learned.

Nina called me the very next day. She said she wanted to try working out. She'd read several articles online about how resistance training could help her, and when she called her doctor to ask his advice, he encouraged her too. Within weeks she felt more flexible and experienced a lot less pain in her joints.

I take a no-excuses approach with my clients. It doesn't mean we can't have valid reasons not to do something, but we must recognize what they are in order to educate ourselves and make the plan to overcome them. Few things are impossible to the willing heart!

TAKE ACTION

. . . .

INVENTORY YOUR EXCUSES

In your B.A.L.A.N.C.E. Journal, list all the excuses you make regarding health, wellness, and weight. Some might be:

- I don't have time to work out.

- The only way to lose weight is to be hungry all the time.

- I can't exercise because I can't afford a gym membership.

- It's impossible for me to lose weight.

- If I could lose 20 pounds, all my problems would be solved and I would be happy.

- It doesn't matter what I eat as long as it's low in calories.

- I don't weight train because I don't want to look like a bodybuilder.

- I don't have time to eat well.

- I can't afford healthful food.

- I have a slow metabolism that won't speed up or change.

- I'm big boned.

- I'm not meant to be thin.

- Healthy food doesn't taste good.

- Overeating helps me feel less stressed.

After you finish your list, hold on to it. We will come back to it later and use it to create successful life and balance strategies.

. . . .

TAKE ACTION

. . . .

FUEL YOUR MIND AS WELL

Choose mind-set fuel that will keep your thoughts aligned with what your heart desires. What fuels our minds and hearts is equally (if not more) important to what we fuel our bodies with. And if we don't choose our fuel sources wisely, we can easily lose our focus. Mind-set fuel includes everything you read, listen to, and watch—the things that feed your brain messages. Let go of the mind-set fuel that brings you down.

Before I move on to this chapter's Everyday B.A.L.A.N.C.E. Technique, I'd like to share with you a journal page from Penny, a woman who took my 30-Day Challenge. Her thoughts about letting go are wonderfully insightful, and I think they may inspire you as you seek to let go of whatever interferes with balance and peace in your life.

I hold on to my old (and often bad) habits like a pair of comfortable sweats. I don't want to let them go. I know the sweats make me look frumpy, ugly. They have stains and holes. But they feel so good! When I wear them, I am free from constriction—I am comfortable.

So too are bad habits. They are comfortable, freeing, and easy to wear. I don't think too much about bad habits; they just happen. Giving them up—or letting go of them—is a wrench. Letting go involves a lot of soul-searching. It's hard, dumping out the detritus of my brain, because it means examining my life—a painful process involving lots of if-only kinds of thoughts.

I must admit, when Jennifer shared the Mind-Set Purification technique, I thought, What the heck! I'm going to start out fresh—who wants to relive the past? But I brain-dumped and figured out something about myself: My unhealthy habits were created in moments of boredom. When I'm engrossed in something, I don't mindlessly reach for the potato chips, the peanuts, or the wine. I have no need to mindlessly eat (and I often simply forget to eat altogether) when I'm writing or gardening—things I love and am passionate about. But when I'm bored, I eat and drink to excess.

What are my boring triggers? Television and chatting on the phone are two major producers of the munchies. So are Facebook and e-mails. Aha!

I need challenges in my life, something to keep my brain active. Never mind about my body, it is my brain that needs to be exercised.

So I dusted off one of the three half-finished novels languishing in my desk drawer and started rewriting one. This keeps me from the morning munchies attack. A session of mind mapping took care of an afternoon munchies attack and gave me ideas of what I want to do with my life.

The only thing left to let go of is my addiction to listening to the news. The world is falling apart, and I feel obligated to take a front-row seat to it all. But because of the stress it causes me, I must cut back. After all, the world did manage very well without me sixty-two years ago. I can't change much; therefore I will let the world get on without my oversight every evening.

It is difficult but necessary to let go. The toxicity of bad habits clogs up my body and life. However, I can't do it all at once. I've got to give myself permission to allow some time to change. One step at a time is the answer, and it is working—slowly, a lot more slowly than I want—but it is working.

There are so many things I wish I'd done. Now is the time to do some of them.

Everyday B.A.L.A.N.C.E. Technique:
Laugh

Being joyful is the best "cosmetic"
I've got in my arsenal of beauty products.
And, the price is right.

—Kara Oh

Laughter comes naturally to children. My little ones are constantly cracking themselves up. They laugh at each other; they laugh at my husband and me; they laugh with their cousins; they laugh at commercials; they laugh and laugh until their bellies hurt. It's adorable, and very contagious.

Most adults laugh less frequently, I've come to realize. This is too bad, because laughter, fun, play, and joy are essential ingredients to being in balance. Without these ingredients, we can lose our creativity, our imagination, and our inner child. Don't say good-bye to that silly little girl inside of you. Reconnect with her—do something completely goofy, laugh out loud, blow some bubbles (without children present), watch a funny movie, get your girl giggle back even for just a few minutes.

Laughter is good for your health. It can increase abdominal strength and help with weight loss. Studies show that thirty minutes of "mirthful laughter" decreases blood levels of the stress hormone cortisol by up to 87 percent!

Prolonged high cortisol levels interfere with the healthy functioning of your thyroid gland as well as your mental performance, bone density, muscle tissue, inflammatory response, and immune system. Excess cortisol can also contribute to blood sugar imbalances, increased body weight, and raised blood pressure.

Laughter boosts immune function, adds oxygen to the blood, stimulates our muscles (that's the best ab workout yet!), and relieves pain.

So take a look at your environment. Does everything about it make you smile? If not, fill your space with happy images, soothing colors, pictures with meaning. Play music, watch movies, tell jokes, pull out old-fashioned games like Twister or Trivial Pursuit, and have a blast at home. Laughing and smiling releases anger and negativity. Simply by having fun, you can live well and improve your health.

Summing Up

In this chapter, we've discussed the tremendous value of undergoing a cleansing process that allows you to let go of the emotional and physical debris that contributes to a life out of balance. Some of the activities I suggested included:

- Do a food cleanse that rids your diet and your kitchen of the foods that serve no good purpose in your life, including fast food, junk food, foods that negatively influence your mood, and foods that trigger overeating.

- Do a cabinet and closet cutback that clears your home of clutter and junk. This process helps you commit to a full-scale change that will bring you closer to finding balance.

- Eliminate time vacuums by evaluating and getting rid of some of the things that unnecessarily suck time out of your life.

- Practice saying no so you can give yourself time and energy to focus on living a healthy, balanced life.

- Take a look at your mind-set and purify it of self-limiting beliefs and unhealthy thoughts that knock you off balance.

In Chapter 5, I'll help you determine the most important things to add to your daily schedule in order to help balance your life and the scale.

Chapter Five

· ·

A is for *Add In* and *Appreciate*

I have a simple philosophy: Fill what's empty.
Empty what's full. Scratch where it itches.

—Alice Roosevelt Longworth

· ·

When I was a little girl, my family and I watched a movie called *Six Weeks*. It is about a twelve-year-old girl named Nicole who is dying from leukemia. She wants to do "one last great thing."

She ends up meeting a politician, and they help each other really live during her final weeks. Nicole skates the ice rink at Rockefeller Center, kisses a boy, dances the lead in *The Nutcracker,* and sightsees in New York City. I loved this movie—it was one of the first times I learned the lesson to live *now*.

Thinking about it recently made me want to write my own bucket list. But I'm not sure I like the term *bucket list*. While I love the idea of having one (and the name is pretty catchy), I think a bucket list may never really come to fruition. Most of us feel immortal, and if we think we have all the time in the world to do these things before we kick the bucket, our goals and dreams may sit in a notebook as we wait for the perfect time to climb our mountains or take our dream vacations. In the movie *Six Weeks,* Nicole knew how much time she had left. In reality, though, we never know. And there may never be a perfect time to start fulfilling the dreams on our bucket list.

Instead of a bucket list, I opted to write a life list—a list of things I want to do now, not sometime in the distant, hazy future. Writing my life list was such an amazing experience. It made me realize that I had the power to add into my life whatever I wanted, that I could enrich it in such a way that was intentional and purposeful. While some things on my life list were extreme—for example, I'd like to anonymously build a home for someone who lost theirs—I realized there are ways that I could add in service like that without having the funding to actually build the home. As I mentioned, I now volunteer with the non-profit organization Enchanted Makeovers, whose mission is to nurture the human connection and to transform shelters into whimsical cottage retreat centers where women and children can live with hope and inspiration. But the only way I could find the time and energy to get involved with this fabulous organization was by going through the process of letting go and adding in.

In the previous chapters we've done a brain dump, made assessments, and let go. When you let go, you made time, energy, and space for new things. Now it's time to add in the new things that will enrich your life and fill you up.

As you begin to add things in, consider the differences between a baker and a cook. A baker measures carefully—a teaspoon of this, a tablespoon of that; every ingredient is added in mindfully and intentionally. But cooking is the exact opposite—you toss in a handful of this, a sprinkle of that. Amounts don't really matter. If you love garlic, you throw in a lot; if you don't, you skip it.

So it is in our lives. We need to add in like bakers, measuring carefully. An extra teaspoon of baking powder can throw an entire cake out of balance. In our lives, even a little too much of one thing can cause an imbalance. Like pebbles on a scale, the little things add up fast. Life will naturally sprinkle things in unexpectedly. Sometimes the sprinkles are fun and surprising, and other times stressful and upsetting. Life is the cook, and we are the bakers. It's up to us to add in with awareness and intention.

How do you know what to add in? One way is to look at the activities you've done so far in this book. The food and diet assessments from Chapter 3 will help you design the best eating plan for you. Time-use assessments, also from Chapter 3, will help you create a schedule that gives you the time you need to meet your obligations, enjoy your life, live healthfully, exercise, take care of yourself, and do the activities you love but thought you didn't have time for. And your excuses inventory from Chapter 4 will help you add in new ways of looking at old excuses.

Before you start adding in, go back to the core values exercise you did in Chapter 2. You can use your core values as a filter to make sure that everything you add in to your life truly reflects your most important values.

I'm not going to tell you exactly what to add in because you need to figure that out for yourself in a way that makes the most sense to you. What you add in will be completely different from what someone else adds in. There are no universal answers, just what's right for you.

As you add things to your life, consider these basics to fuel your heart, mind, and body.

- Choices that honor your core values

- Education

- Movement

- Healthful, nurturing foods

- Time for you

- A support team

Day Design

Doing a day design will help you to tap in to your imagination and open your mind to what you can add into your life. Without limitation, obstacles, or boundaries, I want you to grab your B.A.L.A.N.C.E. Journal and just begin writing ideas for how you would spend your day if you had your complete druthers! Resist the urge to write *shopping* or *maxing out my credit cards* or *sailing away to a deserted island.* I understand you may feel like that at times because of how hectic life can be, but this is about truly designing a day that stirs your soul and makes your spirit soar. Just acknowledging these things can begin the process of opening you up to adding them in.

Choosing what to add in is so important because **action** is what actually creates change. Reading and writing and doing exercises may inspire thought, but our thoughts must be supported by our actions. Otherwise, we can get caught up in a cycle of self-help book after self-help book, diet book after diet book, without ever really making a shift in thinking or being in the world. I'm sure that's never how the author intends it to be, but that's what can end up happening if we don't take the action in our lives.

I am not a huge fan of self-help books for this reason. That probably sounds weird, since I've written a book that may be considered self-help. Let me explain. I want you to find balance, embrace imperfection, and be who you were born to be. I want you to show up in this world, use your gifts, and enjoy life—you deserve that, I deserve that, we all deserve that, even if we were made to believe differently by another human being or experience. I don't believe that anyone is unworthy. We make mistakes, we learn lessons, we heal, we mess up, and we succeed. I feel we are all students and teachers in our lives in different ways. I believe I was born to communicate. I love to listen to and share stories and to inspire and be inspired by others. What I wish for you is that you take action in your life, nurture yourself, and be confident and strong so you can do that which makes you happy and serves others.

In Chapter 4, you read an excerpt from Penny's journal about letting go. When we got to the adding in part of the class, I explained the day design. Penny excitedly went home and began writing all the things she would love to do. She wanted to learn to speak Spanish before her nephew's wedding to a Colombian girl because part of the ceremony would be in Spanish, and many of the guests would be Spanish speakers. She wanted to take a cooking class because she desperately wanted to be more creative with her food. She also wanted to have time to write a novel. Penny was a copywriter, and she spent much of her time writing for others rather than for herself.

As she began to envision her life with these beautiful details, these activities that excited her, she realized she had to let something go to make time to add in these new passions. It occurred to her that my class would be the best thing to let go of! When she told me this, we both had a good laugh. I would miss her, but I agreed completely—like Penny, I would much rather be taking action in my life than *learning about* how to take action in my life. She saw that her learning was done, she was ready, and off she went. I was proud of her—and she promised to buy a copy of this book so she could learn the rest of the techniques!

TAKE ACTION

WHAT WILL YOU ADD IN?

Keep it simple. Begin by writing a list of ten great additions to your daily life and then practicing them one by one. Remember, energy is like an echo: you get back what you put out there. Are you thinking of deprivation or fulfillment? I prefer fulfillment—it's so much more fun than deprivation!

Taking Away vs. Adding In

Sometimes when we are aware that we'd like to make a change, we think about all the things we think we've done wrong or we have to stop doing. I know a lot of people who are just plain old beating themselves up in the name of motivation.

As we discussed in Chapter 4, choosing to let something go can be quite liberating. But if you think you don't have a choice and **must** do something, you may wind up feeling deprived. If you find that you are discouraged and drowning in a take-away mentality, I suggest flipping your focus to what you want to add in to your life vs. what you want to take away. Once you start adding in healthy, happy, authentic behaviors, your body and mind will crave more of them, and as a result, more of them will flow naturally into your life! Let's look at some examples:

Take-away mentality: *I have to give up sweets.*

Add-in mentality: *I will eat more veggies.*

Take-away mentality: *I have to fight less with my partner.*

Add-in mentality: *I will love and communicate better with my partner.*

Take-away mentality: *I have to lose this job and do something I really love.*

Add-in mentality: *I will put passion into whatever I am doing.*

Acknowledging, Honoring, and Activating Your Core Values

In Chapter 2, you assessed your core values. Now is the time to decide how you will honor and activate those values in your daily life and how those values can be woven into the goals you set for yourself.

I've mentioned that core values act as both an anchor and a compass. Let me explain. I know that life can be busy, stressful, exhausting. I understand that completely, and to be quite honest, I used to believe that my happiness and my balance were dependent on my circumstances—the size of my jeans, the state of my love life, and the title on my business card.

Being aware of it now, I realize how crazy it sounds. But I also know many other women subconsciously feel that way too. Whether it's because of messages from the media or relatives or whoever, women who do not have an anchor can easily get thrown way off balance by circumstances. And without our own internal compass guiding us, we can easily go from diet book to diet book to self-help book to self-

B.A.L.A.N.C.E. Tip

Go Back to Bed

If you're not getting enough sleep, you're missing out on a great health booster. Sleep improves mood and memory, contributes to heart health and a strong immune system, reduces stress and anxiety, helps you maintain a healthy body weight, increases your ability to cope with pain, and helps regulate blood sugar. Aim for seven to nine hours a night, keeping in mind that individual sleep needs vary.

help book looking for the way to happiness. By adding in choices that acknowledge your core values, you strengthen your anchor and fine-tune your compass.

While I have many values, my core values are **faith, creativity, inspiration,** and **family.** Just as you have to brush your teeth daily so they don't fall out, you must honor and acknowledge your values daily to keep them strong. So I have daily rituals and visual reminders around each of my core values. I call them my spiritual toothpaste.

For **faith,** I spend time praying and meditating daily. I read a bit of scripture every morning and evening. I tune in to a faith-based radio station during my drive time. And in my family's home, I have several plaques, pictures, and knickknacks that represent my faith. One of the important things for this core value is to take care of not only my spirit but also my body, because it is a gift from God. So I make sure I nurture my body well.

For **creativity,** I spend time each day writing, using my imagination (it's kind of easy to nurture imagination when you have small children), and doing something creative. Whether it's telling my kids a completely made-up-from-my-mind bath-time story, drawing, or making picture collages, each day I do something to honor my value of creativity. On the days I don't honor my creativity, I feel fenced in.

I value creativity with food too. I can't just chomp on celery all day, and the thought of plain anything bores me. I crave flavor! I am a creative foodie crunched for time, so I buy all different kinds of spices, herbs, and pure extracts. With these tools, it's easy to create simple, unique foods. Forget about thirty-minute meals—I specialize in thirty-second meals! Some days I blend up wheat germ, almond milk, pure coconut extract, frozen blueberries, and a pinch of fine shredded coconut, and I feel like I am on a tropical island. Other days, my taste buds take me to a cozy winter cabin so I add cinnamon, nutmeg, pure vanilla extract, and diced warm apples to plain oatmeal. I mash avocado with garlic and lime juice for a burst of flavor that's yummy on just about anything or even simply by the spoon. You can be creative without spending hours on complicated recipes.

For **inspiration,** I like to both inspire and be inspired. In order to acknowledge this value, I have a blog called *Inspired Girl.* I share my personal life lessons and stories in hopes of inspiring my readers, and I interview other inspiring women who share their stories. I also teach classes that inspire and take classes to be inspired. I receive a daily dose of inspiration in my inbox, and I send a daily inspirational message to my e-mail list. It's a circle of inspiration!

When it comes to movement, I honor inspiration as a core value because I know that my personal inside-out transformation inspires others and that movement is key. I work out at Curves because the upbeat music, the friendly circle of women, and the environment all serve as inspiration to me.

For **family,** all my decisions are made with the greater good of my family in the front of my mind. Spending time with my family is incredibly important for me because time and presence are the most precious gifts we can give the people we love. I realize my children may not remember the toys they once had, but they will remember us spending time in the kitchen together, out in the yard climbing trees, or walking on the beach collecting shells. Our photo albums are filled with experiences, not things.

There have been times when I could have worked longer hours to see more clients and earn more income, but I chose not to so I could be home with my family. There are also times when I am required to travel for work, and I know by doing so I am able to provide for my family. On a daily basis, I make sure I spend quality time with my children, speak on the phone with my parents, and drink coffee on the porch with my husband. I consciously value my family, and my decisions are centered on them. It really is all about defining your own meaning and method for balance.

I also know that being a healthy, happy, balanced mom is so important for my family, so I must spend time taking care of me too. When

I am working out or eating fresh, delicious food, I am honoring my **family** value.

TAKE ACTION

. . . .

LET YOUR CORE VALUES GUIDE YOU

Write down each of your core values, and then describe how you can honor and recognize them on a daily basis. Make sure you also think about your life vision and goals, and weave the core values into them as well. If you aren't honoring your values daily (that is, you lack spiritual toothpaste) figure out ways to do just that so your values are strong, your anchor is sturdy, and your compass is pointed in the right direction. And remember, when you let your core values guide you, you won't be as attached to outcomes. You'll feel so good, you'll enjoy the process!

. . . .

Add In Education

Educating yourself may sound boring. But it is so important. The more we truly understand something, the easier it is to implement in our lives. And once we begin understanding, learning becomes more and more invigorating. For example, I used to think nothing of drinking orange juice—who has time to peel and eat an actual orange? Besides, the juice has vitamin C so it's really no different, right? *Wrong!*

When I learned that the digestion process was completely different when you eat an orange versus drinking the juice, it really made me stop and think. The white rind on the orange provides fiber that prepares your body for the sugar in the fruit of the orange. When you bite into the rind, the fiber sends a signal to your body. It aids the digestion of the fruit—something that doesn't happen when you're drinking a carton of processed orange juice.

Because I was prediabetic, I choose to watch my sugar intake carefully. After learning that the full fruit is near perfect in form, from skin to pulp, I made time to eat oranges instead of just drinking juice.

If you're reaching for orange juice instead of soda, it's a healthier option for sure. But the real benefits from fruit often are found in skin and pulp, which is generally absent in juice (even 100 percent fruit juice). My point is this: educate yourself on your options, and then make informed decisions that are best for you.

Learning about food, digestion, and metabolism opened my eyes to the miracles of nature. Whole, natural food is generally perfect by design (when humans don't mess with it too much). I also learned that eating like a bird in order to lose weight actually contributes to gaining weight. When your body is starving, it slows your metabolism down and your body starts to hoard calories.

When I understood that a calorie is not just a calorie—that the quality of my food affects every aspect of my being—I thought differently about merely counting calories or fat grams or carbohydrates. I now opt for high-quality foods to fuel and energize my body and life well.

And of course, I had to learn how to deal with the whole blood sugar spike and dip thing. Wow! When I learned to eat at regular intervals, my blood sugar stabilized and I felt better. For the first time in my life, I could eat foods I loved, feel good, and release weight. That was the end of starvation diets followed by binging fits for me.

Food can dramatically affect the way you feel and act. I once had a boyfriend who was very moody. In a blink of an eye, he would go silent or pick a fight with me. For the most part he was a nice, caring guy, but at different points throughout the week, he would go bad. After a few months with him, I saw the connection: when he went long periods without eating, his mood, demeanor, attitude, and communication style completely changed for the worse.

Our Curves members tell me similar stories about their children, whose attention spans and attitudes are influenced by food. One member's doctor wanted to prescribe medication for her son's behavior problems. Distraught at the idea of medicating such a young child, the woman educated herself and observed her son's actions closely, finding links between his behavior and his eating habits. He ate a big bowl of sugary cereal in the morning, went for hours without a snack, and then had a starchy lunch such as instant pasta or another bowl of sugary cereal. By the time he got home from school, he was a mess. So this member changed her son's diet, feeding him a nutritious breakfast, a healthy mid-morning snack, and a nutritious lunch. His behavior improved, his attention span increased, and his personality came back to life without medications.

I encourage you to empower yourself with education. Understand how your body works, how digestion works, how metabolism works. Don't simply take things at face value—understand for yourself.

Another member said she was giving up on weight loss because of her underactive thyroid. Her knowledge about thyroid issues seemed incomplete, so I suggested she educate herself. She discovered that she was quite misinformed about thyroid health and didn't have to give up on weight loss. She began working her muscles, focusing on strength and muscle development. She learned about foods that promote muscle growth and realized she wasn't eating enough healthy protein. With a little education, she went from depressed and disgusted with her body to energized and empowered with information! And she was clearly prepared to take action by focusing on what she could control, rather than what she could not.

If you were sitting in your living room and the lights went out, what would you do? Probably check the switch and replace the bulb. If those things didn't work, you might check the circuit breaker and, if necessary, call in an electrician. You wouldn't simply sit in the dark or light a candle as a temporary fix. But we often sit in the dark when it comes to our bodies. Turn on the light! Learn as much as you can about your body and the way it functions best.

Add In Movement:
A Complete Cardiovascular and
Strength Training Workout

One of the funniest comics I've ever seen was of two women taking the elevator to the twentieth floor of a building so they could go to a gym to use the stair climber. I laughed out loud when I looked at it, probably because I saw a bit of my (former) self in the comic. Some people are born to work out and love going to the gym. Unfortunately, I wasn't one of those people. I never had the urge to run on a treadmill or pump iron in front of a mirror. I always had to force myself to go to the gym. But once I found exercise I enjoyed, it became easier.

If exercise bores you, it may be because you have been doing the wrong kind of exercise. When choosing an exercise, think about your personality type, your interests, and your core values. Find exercise that activates and honors your core values. Then you'll be more likely to enjoy it!

- If you're spiritual, look for a spiritual workout like yoga, or exercise with someone who shares your spiritual outlook. Walk together and talk about faith. A yoga class may speak to your core values the way a stair climber session doesn't.

- If one of your core values is socializing with others, consider group exercise. I met a woman who struggled with her lone workouts. She found them boring and energy sapping. When she thought about her core values, she realized that having lots of alone time was definitely not on her list. She loved being with people any chance she got! So she signed up for a group exercise class, and her three-times-a-week exercise time went from dull to fun. She quickly made friends, and she enjoyed herself so much she barely realized she was exercising. Her class has parties and goes for occasional hikes after class. A few members even formed a reading group that got together monthly for wine and book talk. Instead of dreading exercise, she can't wait to spend time with these active, exciting women.

Remember that hunky guy from the Diet Coke commercial? His name is Lucky Vanous, and he made an exercise video. I worked out with that video for about six months—every day I had a date with Lucky. I eventually got tired of it—Lucky lost his luster, I guess. But for a while, Lucky was my go-to exercise motivation.

Because I don't naturally enjoy exercise, I really had to search to find something that fit my personality and my core values. I began by going to a traditional gym, and while I loved the people there, I really didn't love spending an hour and a half doing cardio and strength training. Finally, I found something that made me come alive when I walked through the door.

When I first heard about Curves from my coworker Julie, I was skeptical. She and her mother owned a franchise, but they started out as members of another. Julie raved about Curves, but I just couldn't imagine it. She looked incredibly toned, but could a thirty-minute workout really work for me? Would it bore me to death? Despite my misgivings, I gave it a try along with my mom and sister-in-law. We worked out at Julie and Sue's Curves for a couple months, and we were in love with the workout, the community, the size of the facility, and of course, the overall feeling of well-being that came from the Curves philosophy. Julie and Sue watched us as we worked out, showing us how to do the movements properly and effectively. Julie would push me too. She would say, "The circuit only works if you work it!"

We were hooked. I imagined all the women who felt the same as I did and would benefit from this nontraditional workout. Within a year, my mom and I opened a Curves location, and then my sister-in-law opened one too. That was eleven years ago, and we're still working out on the circuit. And Curves has continually reinvented itself to keep women excited about living well—we have CurvesSmart® equipment now, which tells us the specifics of our workout and if we are working out hard enough. We incorporate Curves with Zumba for a little splash of dance-inspired fitness. In 2012, we launched the Curves Complete program, a one-stop shop for wellness and weight loss with nutrition, fitness, and coaching combined.

Bottom line: there are tons of ways to work your muscles and elevate your heart rate. So no excuses! You've got to do it! Find movement that moves you, and go for it.

Beyond Weight Loss

If you've got the dieter's mentality, then you probably think of exercise simply as a way to burn calories. But it's so much more. It really is a necessity for a healthy, balanced life.

Movement and muscle strength are key to longevity. They give you more energy, allow you to burn more calories, and make you feel vibrant. A strong, healthy body is one of the foundations to a strong, healthy life. Exercise does take time. But if you make it an add-in priority, you can most likely fit it in to your life. If not, you may need to let go of other tasks in order to make room for it.

Exercise has so many benefits beyond just burning calories. It also:

- Strengthens your bones

- Improves your mood by releasing endorphins and other natural feel-good chemicals into your blood

- Slows down the normal muscle loss that occurs as you age

- Improves your balance, coordination, and posture

- Increases your metabolism

- Reduces the effects of stress on your body

- Helps keep your blood sugar in check

- Helps relieve pain from arthritis and other ailments

- Helps lower cholesterol, blood pressure, and other heart disease risks

- Boosts blood flow to the brain, which helps you think more clearly

- Reduces your risk of an array of diseases

- Boosts your circulation, which speeds up the body's natural detoxification process

- Increases your energy level

- Helps you sleep better at night

- Improves your libido

So What Do I Do?

Fitness has three components: strength training, cardiovascular training, and stretching. To be truly fit, you have to do all three.

Strength training: If you want to have a higher metabolism, stronger bones, less chronic pain, and more energy—and who doesn't?—you absolutely must work your muscles. I'm not just talking about your arms because they show in a sleeveless shirt or your abdomen because you want a flat bikini belly. This kind of spot toning doesn't work. You've got to work every major muscle group to benefit from strength training.

Cardiovascular training: If you want to rev up your weight loss even more and build heart health, you've got to do exercise that pumps up your cardiovascular system. This doesn't mean walking around your block at a leisurely pace—it means elevating your heart rate to a level that strengthens your heart.

I can't tell you how many women I've worked with who have spent years walking or using the elliptical machine or taking aerobic classes without ever losing weight. The problem is, they didn't push hard enough to elevate their heart rate. If you aren't

Estimated Target Heart Rate by Age

To give your heart a workout, you've got to get your heart rate up into what's called the target heart rate range. Target heart rate is calculated by first determining your maximum heart rate (220 minus your age) and multiplying it by 0.50 for the low end of the range and 0.85 for the high end. No need to do any math, though—here's a chart that tells you your range.

Age	Target Heart Rate Range (beats per minute)
20	100–170
25	98–166
30	95–162
35	93–157
40	90–153
45	88–149
50	85–145
55	83–140
60	80–136
65	78–132
70	75–128

Source: American Heart Association

elevating your heart rate, you aren't strengthening your heart muscle. This is one of the very important things I learned at Curves, where participants are taught to monitor their heart rate at least three times during a workout.

Stretching: Gently stretching your muscles improves tone, maintains elasticity, increases flexibility, expands range of motion, and helps reduce risk of injuries. Done correctly, it can also make you feel great! You can incorporate stretching into your fitness routine or take yoga or other classes that emphasize stretching. Be sure to get expert stretching advice, either from an exercise book, a trainer, or a fitness class instructor, because performing stretches incorrectly can cause harm. The general rule with stretching is to stretch until you feel a gentle pull but never to the point of discomfort, or you risk muscle tears.

As far as your workout length is concerned, experts have different opinions. I believe a quick, high-quality workout is far better for your body than a long, low-quality one. Just going through the motions of strength training or doing cardiovascular movement is not enough. To get the most from your workout, focus on high-quality exercise that challenges your body and tires you out.

Add In Foods That You Love, That Nurture You, and That Fill You Up

In case you haven't already noticed, I'll just say it: I love food! I am a foodie through and through, and I definitely do not believe that we should deprive ourselves of enjoying food. I love food so darn much, I married a chef. It was a prerequisite for the guys I dated: if they didn't love food or know how to cook, they were out. I am serious about loving and enjoying food.

To begin adding in your favorite foods, do a **brain dump** and list them all in your B.A.L.A.N.C.E. Journal. Include every last chip, candy bar, and rich sauce, even if your dieter's mentality labels them as bad foods. Get it all on paper. If you love pizza, write it down. Chicken francaise, Chinese fried rice, cheesecake, French toast, waffles with syrup, eggplant Parmesan, barbecue potato chips, chocolate chip cookies—acknowledge what you love. Then you can begin to figure out ways to make a healthy and delicious version of the same flavors and textures.

For example, if you love pizza, it doesn't make sense to decide that you'll never eat it again just because it's high in calories and fat. That is unrealistic, and it's also not necessary. You can figure out ways to make pizza as healthy as possible so you can eat it every week and enjoy it. One of my clients chooses flatbread pizza because it is much lower in carbohydrates and calories than doughy pizza. Another pulls off half the cheese. Another has her favorite loaded pizza but eats only one slice instead of her usual three or four.

I believe that people love the flavors and textures of their favorite foods, not necessarily the food itself. I used to say I loved peanut butter cups. But I realized I actually loved the combination of chocolate and peanut butter together in a compact bite. So when I'm craving a peanut butter cup, I choose instead to have a dark chocolate square with a smudge of peanut butter. It satisfies my desire for peanut butter and chocolate in a much healthier way.

One of my absolute favorite flavors is coconut. During a trip to the Turks and Caicos Islands a few years back, I discovered that I adore coconut-crusted chicken and fish. I had to figure out a way to make coconut-crusted food a staple, but in a healthy way. So after a little trial and much error, I came up with a Caribbean-inspired, delicious, healthy, and super-simple meal. Instead of dipping the chicken in whole eggs, I combine two egg whites with one whole egg and add a splash of pure coconut extract. This way, I get an extra flavor of the coconut. For the crust, I mix Panko bread crumbs with finely shredded coconut. A finer shred of coconut allows me to use less and eliminate about 40 percent of the calories and fat. I also bake it in the oven instead of frying. It is coconut-crusted deliciousness!

I have met many women who say they absolutely couldn't live without sausage—they love the spicy flavor and the texture. I suggest textured vegetable protein, a soy product that is much healthier than sausage. This versatile, high-protein food easily takes on other flavors and can substitute for meat in many dishes. It's simple to make: just sauté some in a pan with veggies and spices. When sausage lovers try it, they are shocked—some like it even more than sausage!

Next take a look at your Food Assessment Worksheet in Chapter 3. What's missing from your usual daily diet? Some of my clients realize they eat *zero* vegetables (iceberg lettuce on a Big Mac doesn't count). They eat no dark, leafy greens or colorful yellow, orange, or red fruits and vegetables, all of which are bursting with cancer-fighting antioxidants and loads of other great nutrients. Looking back, I can't believe I was one of those people too.

Add in healthy, nutritious, filling foods—vegetables, fruits, legumes, whole grains. Often when you add in these foods, the less healthy foods drop out of your diet naturally because you're too full to eat them!

You may also notice from your Food Assessment Worksheet that you aren't eating satiating foods, that the calories seem empty and don't really fill you up. If so, try adding in satiating whole grains. For breakfast, choose oatmeal with diced peaches or scrambled eggs on whole-grain toast. Enjoy a bowl of carrot and cashew soup between lunch and dinner. Fish—especially thick, white fish—is high on the satiety index, so cut it into kebabs, toss it on the grill with some vegetables, and serve over brown rice for a filling meal.

Also, consider whether there was something you enjoyed from a past diet that makes sense to add in. Perhaps you loved the Sassy Water recipe from Flat Belly Diet—if you enjoyed it and it fits your healthy, balanced lifestyle, add it in!

As you add food back into your diet, ask yourself these simple questions:

1. Does this food choice **fuel** my body with healthy, pure ingredients or nutrients?

2. Does this food choice elevate my **mood** before, during, and after I eat it?

3. Does this food choice boost my **energy** level in a positive way?

4. Does this food choice give me **simple pleasure** before, during, and after eating?

5. Do I **feel good** about this food choice? If not, is there a way to create a healthier version for everyday purposes or to cut the portion?

6. Can I make a **simple switch** with this food choice (examples may be regular milk to 2% or skim, flavored sugary yogurt to plain nonfat yogurt with fresh berries tossed in, hamburger on a processed bun to a burger wrapped in lettuce)?

7. Is this choice a **beloved comfort food** (for example, macaroni and cheese), or does it represent a deep-rooted family **tradition** (lasagna, kugel, or baklava)? If so, does it serve my body and life well? If not, is there a way to create a healthier version, to eat smaller portions, or to have it less often?

If a food serves no valuable purpose, think twice before adding it back in. You may feel better without it.

Sample Grocery Shopping List

Creating a grocery list at home gives you time to make smart choices about which foods you'll add into your diet. Having a list in hand also saves time and money. I can't tell you what to buy, but I will share with you a thoughtfully devised grocery list from one of the women in my 30-Day Challenge groups. It may help you create a list that works for you.

Grains	Canned/Jarred Items
Oat Cereal	White Beans
Brown Rice	Diced Tomatoes
Steel-Cut Oatmeal	Olive Tapenade
Small 100% Whole-Wheat Pitas	Hummus
Couscous	Almond Butter
Wasa Crackers	Pumpkin Butter
Ak-Mak Crackers	*(continued)*

Nuts

Raw Walnuts

Raw Almonds

Chopped Pistachios

Spices/Baking

Olive Oil

Canola Oil

Sea Salt

Pepper

Apple Cider Vinegar

Cinnamon

<70% Cocoa Dark Chocolate Bar

Pure Vanilla Extract

Pure Almond Extract

Pure Coconut Extract

Dark Baker's Cocoa

Dairy/Refrigerated

Skim Milk

Light Almond Milk

Eggs

Finely Shredded Part-Skim
    Mozzarella Cheese

Plain Greek Low-Fat Yogurt

Part-Skim Ricotta Cheese

Low-Fat Cottage Cheese

Chicken/Turkey/Fish

Skinless, Boneless Chicken
    Breasts

Salmon

Tuna

Tilapia

Frozen Foods

Frozen Unsweetened
    Raspberries, Strawberries,
    and Blackberries

Health Food Aisle

Soy or Whey Protein

Flaxseed

Produce

Classic Romaine Lettuce

Dark, Leafy Lettuce

Asparagus

Broccoli

Cauliflower

Mushrooms

Red Onions

Zucchini

Apples

Spaghetti Squash

Yams

Tomatoes

Green Beans

Eggplant

Edamame

Garlic

Fresh Parsley, Basil, and
    Rosemary

Ginger

Lime

Avocado

Fresh Raspberries

Fresh Blueberries

Grapefruit

Add In Passion, Zest, and Zeal for Life: The Most Beautiful Woman in the World . . . Is YOU!

I am taking a stand against women feeling *less than* because of their size, hair color, financial situation, or relationship status. I think a woman who just plain old loves life is the most beautiful woman in the world.

I know what it's like to feel *less than*—I've been there and could probably write an entire book about that topic. But it would be B-O-R-I-N-G! The bottom line is that you don't need to look a certain way, wear a certain label, hold a certain job title, or have a certain someone in order to be absolutely beautiful from the inside out. You don't even need to have found your purpose.

There is one way to instantly glow, and that is to put passion into everything you do. Then your purpose will unfold naturally, and you won't have to work like a bull to figure it out. People will come into your life because your passion and love for life will bring them to you. You will take care of yourself because you love yourself and we nurture what we love.

I am inspired by many women, all of whom share this one thing in common: they are passionate about life. These are the women who rock in my book. And this is (in essence) the definition of an inspirista. So today, put *love* into everything you do, say, and see. Judge nothing, not even yourself. Look at the world through a passionate lens!

Here are three simple steps to adding in passion, zest, and zeal for life:

1. **Look within.** You don't have to leave happiness up to chance— you have the power to be your best self every single day. In your B.A.L.A.N.C.E. Journal, answer these simple questions to identify how you can be your best self:

- When are you smiling and laughing the most? Describe exactly what you are doing, where you are, who you are with.

- Are you being realistic? In other words, does the image of you as your best self fit? Is it the woman you are today? Does it fit in your world and your reality? If not, start again with question 1.

- How can you incorporate this on a daily, weekly, or more regular basis?

2. **Take advantage of the little *you* moments.** Little *you* moments are the opportunities you have throughout your day to pamper yourself in small but meaningful ways. They include the way your space is designed, the music you listen to in the car, the lotions and face wash you use, the scent of your shampoo, the weekly at-home spa treatments you give yourself. Little *you* moments are the best, and they fit seamlessly into your life! By taking advantage of little *you* moments, you are practicing self-care at a proactive, preventive level.

   Self-care on a **preventive** level helps keep you feeling balanced even when life is hectic, stressful, and exhausting. Then when a big stressor comes along, you're better prepared for it.

3. **Have regular date nights.** Every girl needs a date night every now and then. It doesn't have to be romantic—it just needs to get you away from the stresses of everyday life and make you smile. You can date your spouse, your friends, your sister, your entire family, or even yourself. Do whatever is fun—go out or stay in. Go to a restaurant with pals. Or stay home, run a bath, light a candle, pour your favorite drink, and read a book. If you and the girls haven't gone clubbing in decades, hit the club and dance it up. If you and your husband crave a night out but don't have much time or money to spare, make a mini-date—converse over coffee at a dimly lit café, grab a glass of wine and listen to

music, share an appetizer at your favorite restaurant. It will be quick, but it's just enough time to connect.

Date nights should happen regularly and be built right in to your schedule. If weekly date nights are impossible, make them biweekly or once a month. The important relationships in our lives should never suffer because of lack of time, so make it a point to get together as often as realistically possible. Date nights can be spontaneous or planned. The only rule is that they have to be fun. Here are some examples:

- Create a carpet picnic in the living room and surprise someone special. Go all out and include a picnic basket, flowers, wine, and dessert.

- View the night sky from a mountain, hill, or beach. Lie on the ground and look at the moon. Bring a map of the constellations on a clear night and search away.

- Get lost! Fill up your gas tank, turn on the tunes, and take a mini road trip to nowhere. Explore a town you are unfamiliar with and find a spot to eat, walk, and learn about the town's history from some locals.

- Support talent in your town. Many local bars, restaurants, bookstores, galleries, and libraries invite artists, musicians, or writers to share their talent. Check out your newspaper or go online to find something unique happening in your own backyard.

- Dress to the nines for no reason! You may have a gown sitting in your closet that you've only worn once. I'm sure your friends may too! Plan a girls' night out or take your mate on a date. You don't have to go for fancy food—you can walk around town window shopping, go to a boardwalk, or just hit a local coffee shop.

- Take a cooking class or hire a chef (or culinary school apprentice) to come to your home and give a private cooking lesson. It sounds extravagant, but you may be able to find student chefs willing to do this just for the experience of cooking and teaching.

Picture Yourself as a Goddess

We are bombarded with unrealistic images of beauty and bodies. In the media, cellulite—which almost every woman has—is erased, abdominal muscles are added, skin is made flawless, and hair is always perfect. These unrealistic standards make it difficult for us to feel good and to love ourselves, and they often lead us down the destructive path of dieting, feeling *less than,* and going to unhealthy lengths in the name of looking good.

Enter inspirista Jessica Morrisy, who shoots Goddess Boudoir Photography. Jessica is an advocate of feeling confident and beautiful at any size. She has a gift for making women feel comfortable and shooting absolutely gorgeous photos of them. As Jessica says, "Each woman is a goddess, even if she doesn't always feel like one!"

Jessica's photographic style evokes that feeling within—making a woman feel sexy, classy, confident, and empowered. It is her dream to give this gift to each woman she photographs, so I asked her to share some tips to help us all feel like this. After putting some of her tips into action, I feel more connected to my femininity, and a photo shoot with her only increases that feeling. I strongly suggest you get your own professional photograph taken.

Here are some of Jessica's tips:

Mirror matters: Our minds are the single most powerful tool when it comes to feeling beautiful. When we look in the mirror, typically we notice the things we don't like about ourselves: the creases on our forehead, the pimples on our cheeks, the dimples on our bottom. Instead, use your mirror to focus on the things you love about yourself: the sparkle in your eyes, the whiteness of your teeth, the soft curl of your hair, the arch of your foot. Get a full-length mirror at a craft store and use it just for this purpose. Buy a red or pink lipstick and write the things you love about yourself on the mirror. Gaze at the positive, and forget the other stuff. You'll feel beautiful in no time!

Simple indulgences: Pull out that stemware that's collecting dust, pour yourself a glass of something special, and grab some strawberries or a single chocolate truffle. Or turn on your iPod and dance to your favorite music! There's something to be said for these simple pleasures, and it shouldn't take a special occasion or a certain size in our clothing or even a significant other to bring them to us. By doing these things on your own regularly, you will feel empowered, strong, confident, and truly goddess-like.

Snap a shot: Goddess Boudoir Photography is all about bringing out your inner goddess and embracing your beauty as a woman. It can be challenging to see yourself as gorgeous, but taking the time to treat yourself to a special photo shoot can completely change the way you perceive yourself. Each time you view the images, you can reignite your inner goddess!

TAKE ACTION

BRAINSTORM LITTLE *YOU* MOMENTS

Do a brain dump that lists ways to turn ordinary moments into little *you* moments. For example:

- Create a spa in the shower with special scented soap and a fluffy white washcloth.
- Wear comfy slippers around the house.

- Use high thread count sheets.

- Choose a meaningful mug for sipping morning tea or coffee.

- Wake up fifteen minutes early and spend time reading, meditating, stretching, or just being before the day's chaos begins.

- Make a mixed CD or special iPod playlist with your favorite tunes to listen to while driving or working out.

- Use a special oil treatment for your hair and let it soak in while you do laundry or other household duties.

- Rub essential oils into your temples.

- Lube your legs with your favorite lotion.

- Do something completely silly while cleaning the house.

- Eat your lunch on a blanket in the grass.

- Take a warm milk bath.

B.A.L.A.N.C.E. Tip

Break Out That Smile

Smiling has many benefits to your overall health and well-being. It can actually boost your mood, and it is contagious, so it helps boost others' moods as well. It relieves stress and helps the immune system work better. It releases endorphins, serotonin, and other feel-good compounds in the body. When you smile, your mind is sharper and your awareness is heightened. You work better, and your relationships improve. You are your best self. The power in a simple smile really is amazing!

Nicole's Balanced Beauty Basics

Inspirista Nicole Lundy is the founder of Ne'Lani Beauty and is known as a beauty expert for the modern woman juggling life. She helps women who are going through major life transitions put their best face forward when stress is high and pressure is on.

I know what being busy can do to a beauty routine—I admit I used baby wipes to clean my face for almost two years after having my children. I am a little embarrassed even admitting it, because I know better. Not having time should have been **no excuse** to neglect the largest organ of my body. Even though I was eating well, my skin was drier and my pores were clogged. I adore Nicole—she understands that women are busy, so she thinks up simple ways for us to take care of ourselves. Here are three of Nicole's Balanced Beauty Basics:

1. **Cleanse.** Skin care is the foundation of our beauty, and it is important that we practice a routine morning and night. By practicing a proper routine (no matter how quick it is), your skin will respond to the positive changes and the care you are taking of it. Begin simply. If you have no routine at all, try a five-second wipe down with a warm cloth and cleanser, followed by a dab of moisturizer. If you are doing the minimal, take it up to the two-minute skin care routine: use a good cleanser, circle it on your skin for a minute, rinse well with cool water, and finish with a moisturizer and one-minute face massage. And if you've been doing the two-minute deal, splurge on a five-minute skin care routine: begin with a warm towel on your face for thirty seconds to open up your pores, circle in cleanser for a minute and a half, rinse well with cool water, swipe on toner after cleansing, and finish off with moisturizer and a ninety-second face massage.

2. **Balance.** Wearing makeup can feel like an ordeal, and many of us avoid it. Or we feel like we need it desperately and go way

overboard, which takes away from our natural beauty and can wreak havoc on our skin if we don't have a great cleansing routine. I say, find balance with your makeup routine. Don't hide behind it—just use it to feel polished and pretty. When you feel polished and pretty, your confidence soars, you smile more, and you take care of yourself inside and out. Here are three routines for three different time constraints:

- Five seconds: Apply mascara and lipstick

- Two minutes: Apply concealer, define eyebrows, and apply mascara and lipstick

- Five minutes: Smooth on foundation, define eyebrows, and apply eye shadow, liner, blush, mascara, and lipstick

Many women don't know what colors to pick, or they're wearing the same makeup they wore in 1982. I suggest taking a trip to the beauty counter at one of your favorite department stores on a slow day or evening. Ask someone whose makeup you admire to help you pick out some colors. Most makeup artists love helping people feel gorgeous and would be more than happy to match you up with perfect shades, even if you don't purchase them. They may even write a custom color sheet for you. If the makeup is too expensive, take note of the colors and find a less expensive version.

3. **Hydrate.** For beautifully natural, dewy skin, try coconut water. This super-hydrator, which is rich in minerals, potassium, and electrolytes, helps you to flush out toxins and absorb nutrients to give you a healthy glow from within. Drink it instead of one of your daily water servings.

Add In a Support System:
Enlist the Troops and Build a Team

My husband was an athlete in high school. He played football, and he often tells me stories about the good old days with the guys. He had an incredible coach and assistant coach as well as a whole team of people who worked together with common goals in mind: to win, to play the sport well, and to learn something from every game.

As in sports, we are all more likely to succeed if we have a team of supportive people working with us to achieve a common goal. That's especially true with health, releasing weight, and being in balance: support encourages success.

Many women have support teams for finances, accounting, legal issues, events such as weddings, and even for their hair and nails. But for some reason, many women choose to go through personal change alone. Then they wonder why it's so difficult. I get it! I used to do that too.

I Am Here

Support is one of the best predictors of success, especially when it comes to making health-related changes. There are two basic types of support we need when making a life change: **support of knowledge** (information, examples, education, action) and **support of people** (family, friends, groups, coaches, health care providers).

Support of knowledge: You're reading this book, so you're already educating yourself and are in the process of self-discovery. I encourage all my clients to always continue acquiring knowledge. Read books, take courses, ask questions, and listen to other people's stories. Constant learning is one of the best ways to stay connected with your goals.

Most wellness professionals will tell you the reason they are so committed to living well and teaching others how to do so is the knowledge they have about the subject. Just knowing that every-day choices like how much we move or what we eat can affect our entire being (from mood to energy levels to state of health to confidence to relationships), it's near impossible to choose anything but health. This knowledge not only comes from continual coursework and reading, but also from working with people who have a similar mission to be healthy. This is one of the reasons I believe that when we teach what we once most needed to learn, it reinforces our education and keeps us connected to our personal goals, so we can be who we were born to be.

Support of people: I know firsthand how important it is to have the support of people. My family and friends are an integral support team in my life. I also have a professional support team of colleagues, mentors, and networking groups. Each of my supporters serves a somewhat different role in my life. Of course, I have my husband and our parents, who are supportive no matter what. I call my friend Ellen when I need a voice of reason. My sister-in-law, Danielle, listens, questions, and helps come up with solutions; and there's Jess, who's practically like a younger sister! She listens without judgment—she loves me, flaws and all. My dear friend Marta is also a supporter, or Terry, who has a strong anchor in faith, and they always say just the right words. For business issues, I turn to my Savor the Success mastermind group or online community—these women rock! Not only in business issues but also in helping work through challenges or simply savoring our success together—their support is incredible. When I set a goal, I usually find a mentor or coach to support me through the process. Knowing who to go to for what type of support I need eliminates a whole bunch of time I would spend calling everyone I know and rambling.

Before I make a phone call or enlist a supporter, I take a beat just to listen to my heart. Sometimes the need to reach out to someone goes away and I find peace within. Other times, I reach out to the person in my mental Rolodex who can give me the type of support I need.

Support can come from family, friends, coworkers, an online group, a health center, a group exercise class, or a personal coach, just to name a few. Believe it or not, I found a great supporter just by frequenting the same Dunkin' Donuts (for coffee, of course) daily.

We can read books, take courses, and fill out worksheets, but we *must* complement this knowledge with what we learn from the actions and experiences of others—not from their preaching, but from their stories, choices, and the example of how they live.

Parents are a great example of this. A mother may tell her child to be kind to others. But this lesson is far more meaningful when a child observes her mother's kindness in action. We are in a constant state of teaching and learning just by being. If you want to teach people joy, you must be joyful—and by being joyful, you are learning joy. If you want to teach people strength, you must be strong, and then you are learning strength.

Supporters are people who hold you in their highest regard. They see you as your best self and love you even when you are your worst. If a friend or relative is constantly focusing on your perceived negative qualities and never shining a light on your strengths, this person may not be your first choice as a supporter.

TAKE ACTION

FORM YOUR TEAM

In your B.A.L.A.N.C.E. Journal, make a list of people in your life who lift you up. This could include your spouse, parents, family, friends, or any combination of them. Then expand your view to a pastor at church or a rabbi at temple, a neighbor who always says hello, or a dear co-worker. It could be someone you chat with online, a former teacher, or someone you admire from afar. Once you identify your supporters and mentors, you may want to formalize the relationship and ask them to be part of your support team.

The keys with enlisting the support of people is to first clarify your definition of support and then to take the leap and ask people to become your supporters.

I've worked with many women who say they are surrounded by unsupportive people. I understand. But I believe there are many people who genuinely want to see you succeed at what you set out to do. They just may not know how to do that. We all have different definitions of support, and we certainly can't expect people to know ours unless we articulate it to them. Communication and clarity are crucial. Once you set up support guidelines, you may be shocked at just how supportive the people in your life can be.

Here are some tips to keep in mind while you form your support team:

Be clear about what you're asking for. If you don't communicate the fact that you are looking for support, friends and family may choose to stay silent. For example, if you tell your husband you are trying to lose weight, he may think you don't want to hear anything from him, so he will keep his mouth shut! People sometimes don't want to overstep, so make sure whoever you are putting on your support team knows (and accepts) that they are enlisted.

Be clear about what kind of support you need. How do you feel best supported? For example, you may tell your friend that you want to release some weight. Once she has agreed to support you, she may think the best way to do this is to point out when you're eating something she thinks you shouldn't. This won't help if you hate being monitored by food police. So be clear and communicative about your goals and what your expectation or need for support is. Support can be physical: you may find it helpful to have a supporter go food shopping or walking with you. Support can also be emotional: you may find it beneficial to have someone you can discuss your challenges and successes with. Support can also be encouragement: ideally, your supporters will inspire and encourage you with kind words, praise, and observations. For example, you may want your supporters to notice little things you are doing differently and compliment you on the changes you've made.

Understand that not everyone can be an effective supporter for you. Often people try to be supportive, but even when you clearly explain your goals, they can't give you what you need. That's okay. People who love you can't necessarily support you in the way you want or need. Be grateful, acknowledge their efforts, and recognize that you may need to enlist a different supporter.

I worked with a woman whose mother tried so hard to support her. No matter how many times she told her mother she didn't want her to focus on the calories she ate or the number on the scale, her mother couldn't help herself. One day it turned into a huge argument. My client felt awful. Her mother felt hurt. I advised my client to recognize her mother's efforts but not to expect her mother to change her own ingrained dieter's mentality. Then my client chose to enlist support from her cousin, even though they hadn't talked in a while. Her cousin was happy to hear from her and was quite willing to take over as her chief supporter. My client still spoke with her mother regularly, and because she was receiving the support she needed elsewhere, she could let go of being continually frustrated by unmet expectations and begin to appreciate her mother for who she was.

Show gratitude to your supporters. Thank them for their support, encourage them in their endeavors, and offer to be a member of their support team in return.

☼ Go from Dreaming to Being

Here are two mind-set shifts that can catapult us from dreaming about doing something to being the person we were born to be.

See yourself as you want to be—now. We live up to the expectations and the image we hold for ourselves. We must see and believe that we are complete, whole, capable, resourceful individuals. If you have an intention, phrase it in the present tense. Replace passive, wishful phrases ("I wish I could succeed") with active, strong statements ("I *am* successful!"). Wishing opens the door to feeling bad about your current state, and that negative energy drags you down. Instead, stop wishing and live your vision *now*.

Let your actions speak louder than words. Our actions don't always reflect our goals. Think of a guy who says he wants to settle down and get married, but spends every night at bars flirting with different women. He sends himself and the world a mixed signal. Your thoughts absolutely must align with your actions. Awareness is key. Identify the mixed signals you're sending, either in thought or speech. Write them down, cross them out, and replace them with statements that are in the present tense and that align with your desires.

Everyday B.A.L.A.N.C.E. Technique:
Appreciate

Go to the Everyday B.A.L.A.N.C.E. Techniques when you are in a pinch or when you feel you are overly stressed, exhausted, on the verge of a meltdown, or just getting over a big, bad blowup. These techniques can center you and naturally bring you to a balanced place. Over time, the need to consciously go to them decreases—you begin to use them unconsciously as you benefit from a new way to respond to stress.

There are so many things to appreciate—who you are, friends and family, important objects, circumstances, and events. I even believe it's important to appreciate the curveballs in your life—things that are annoying, hurtful, inconvenient, or bad in any other way.

In a moment of stress, close your eyes and visualize what you appreciate about yourself, others, something in your life, or a circumstance. You may decide to dedicate a section in your B.A.L.A.N.C.E. Journal to appreciation, where you can start listing the life aspects that you appreciate.

When one of my clients did this, she began with the obvious: her family, her friends, and her job. But then she went deeper and added things like: the smell of fresh laundry, the curl in my hair that I tried for years to get rid of, and the way my husband always makes sure the car has gas in it so I am never surprised by an empty tank. Her appreciation list grew and grew, and soon had hundreds of entries. Now, in her moments of frazzle, she looks at the list, focuses on what she has written, and sometimes even adds to it! Her stress levels have plunged, and her joyful feelings have mushroomed.

In my own life, too, the power of appreciation and gratitude is priceless. I am feeling kind of overwhelmed with gratitude at the moment, especially taking this moment to stop and think about the past year—just to name a few:

- My children have grown in leaps and bounds. LuLu is writing, spelling, and reading and is now in school. She is a Daisy Girl Scout. And the Little Man is singing full songs, doing simple addition, and using the computer all by himself. I'm grateful for the way they play together. Yes, there is fighting, but there's also "Sista, you my hero" with her responding, "Oh brother, you're *my* hero!" And those moments make up tenfold for the wrestling on the floor.

- My husband is working so hard to provide for us, not just mone-
tarily, but in so many ways, from helping with all the household
stuff to surprising me with an iced coffee on a long day to being
a kid at heart as he jumps and runs in the leaves with Lu and
the Man. We may sometimes still be on Mars and Venus, but we
always kiss each other goodnight.

- My parents are so amazing. They would do anything for anyone, and they are always willing to lend a hand or an ear, give
encouragement, and believe in us. Their unwavering faith is
such a blessing, and I am so grateful. From driving down at
a moment's notice when something comes up to surprising me
with a beautiful card, everything they do is from the heart. And
even though my parents worry about me still (they are the first
ones I have to call whenever I land in a plane), I've learned to
appreciate their concern.

- My mother-in-law is always thinking of us too. She does so
many little things, and we are lucky to have her kind, generous
heart. She raised her kids on her own, worked very hard all her
life, and instilled that in my husband. I know he is the man he
is because of his mother, and I am so thankful.

Appreciating the Curveballs
and Imperfections

Appreciating life's curveballs is harder than giving thanks for the
blessings, but it's so worthwhile to appreciate the storm that destroyed
your fence, the fact that you were laid off, or your neighbors who constantly get on your nerves.

You're probably thinking, *Why in the world would I appreciate the
bad things that have happened in my life?* In my view, everything

happens for a reason—even the bad things. And very often, the bad ends up leading to good.

My grandmother passed away almost eight years ago. It feels like yesterday, yet it also feels like a lifetime ago. My LuLu and Little Man and Niecey weren't even with us yet, and my husband and I were just friends at that time. My grandmother was amazing. She was a ballroom dancer who danced as long as her lungs allowed her to.

No matter how old I got, when I was in my grandmother's kitchen, I always felt like a little girl playing dress up as I donned her 1920s frocks, put on her pink Mary Kay lipstick, sang songs, and danced with her on the white tile floor.

She was a vibrant, positive woman who loved dragonflies. When her much younger friends would come over and complain about the usual stuff, my grandmother would say, "C'mon, ladies!" and push a button on her plastic flower pot that would sing and dance. She was the original inspirista.

The day my grandmother moved into hospice, family and friends gathered around her. The doctor said she had a few weeks left. That night, my mother and I stayed by her side. While my grandmother slept, my mom and I took turns getting coffee and vending machine snacks, crying, laughing, and talking. Early that morning, my grandmother passed away while my mom and I held her hands.

The sadness paralyzed me. I felt my back stiffen, and for three days I could barely move. The next few days were a blur. At the time, I had several guy friends whom I casually dated, but the only one who showed up at the wake and funeral was Michael. He and I were just friends, but his support in being there for me during a messy, uncomfortable, real-life moment made me see him for his heart. He even delivered a platter of food to my parents. Shortly after that, we began dating.

Almost a year later, Michael and I were married. Then in April, our LuLu (her full name is Millana in honor of my beautiful, strong, inspiring Grandma Millie) was born. Two years later, our Little Man came into the world and was photographed by my dear friend Jessica. In my favorite photo, he is hugging my husband's arm at the tattoo of all our names wrapped around a dragonfly.

Millana is now six and a half. She often sings, and today, she made up a song about dancing. I pictured my grandmother and remembered the song that we played at our wedding for her, "I Hope You Dance."

I feel blessed by the beautiful imperfections that have happened in my life. They gave me strength and taught me so much more than any book alone can teach.

Often there are reasons for circumstances that we simply do not understand. I love to go back and connect the dots, tracing the good things that came as a result of the bad. Just knowing that allows me to have a greater appreciation for the cruddy things while they are happening.

TAKE ACTION

QUESTIONS OF APPRECIATION

I recently chatted with Susan Vernicek, the self-esteem expert as well as founder and editor of *Identity Magazine*, about her take on why appreciation is such an important part of our journey toward loving and nurturing ourselves.

"When we learn to appreciate," she says, "we learn to not take life or what each of us has to offer to this world for granted. It increases our self-esteem so that we no longer think we have to be somebody else, but rather simply be who we are, so we can achieve our personal best. By doing this, we actually become happier," Susan explains.

Appreciation is the bedrock on which self-esteem rests, she adds. "I always say, 'smile to inspire.' But without having appreciation, many women can't even muster up a smile. Many would say they appreciate their friends, family, and certain life experiences that teach valuable les-

sons. I believe we need to first appreciate ourselves before we can appreciate others and our lives."

Susan created the Identity 5 Workshop, which asks women to answer
five key questions about appreciating their identity. "Women are finding
it therapeutic to write down and share what they appreciate about themselves first, then about their lives and those involved in their lives. Many
of us are too busy to slow down and appreciate. The Identity 5 gives you
permission to stop what you are doing and acknowledge who you are
as well as what you are offering yourself, family, friends, colleagues, and
the world."

Here are Susan's Identity 5 questions. Spend some time answering
them in your B.A.L.A.N.C.E. Journal and you'll develop a much better
awareness of the benefits of appreciation in your life.

1. What have you accepted within yourself and within your life,
    mentally and/or physically? Is there anything you are still work-
    ing to accept?

2. What have you learned to appreciate about yourself and your
    life? Is there anything you are still working on appreciating?

3. What have you achieved? (This accomplishment can be anything
    that *you* are most proud of.) What have you achieved that has
    made you smile cheek to cheek? What are you still working to
    achieve?

4. What is your not-so-perfect way? We are all unique with quirks
    and imperfections, so why not flaunt them and embrace them?
    These imperfections create your character and your identity.
    (Note: If you find that you are just listing negative traits of your-
    self, dig deeper.)

5. How would you complete the sentence, " I love my . . ."? Nine
    out of ten women list what they love in life—family, friends, or
    work—but this is about *you*. So refrain from answering about

others and focus on what you love about yourself mentally and physically, and then within your life.

Beth is a wonderful woman who experienced six years of childhood sexual abuse. Notice her strength and authenticity in the way she answered the Identity 5 questions.

1. I will no longer accept crumbs from people. I did that for so many years. I have learned how to have boundaries and to no longer give-give-give in the hopes that someone will throw me a crumb of love. I am working on accepting the limits that my body is beginning to have. I have developed arthritis, and I miss the feeling of running, but my feet can't do it anymore.

2. I appreciate being surrounded by people who love and accept me the way I am, and I appreciate that I am incredibly blessed and lucky to have survived the journey through recovery.

3. I have achieved becoming a published author and knowing that my books provide comfort and peace to people. They're fiction, not self-help, but a lot of people who have been abused find hope in reading Ashley's story. (Ashley is the name of the protagonist in *The Patience Trilogy*).

4. We are all unique with quirks and imperfections, so why not flaunt them and embrace them! I do so struggle with my weight. I have an eating disorder and body dysmorphia too—which means I see my body according to how well I'm managing my eating disorder. I struggle with feeling shame at having regained some of the weight I'd lost.

5. I love my creativity and ability to write. It's really cool!

For more amazing stories and Identity 5 appreciation answers from some incredible women, go to www.identitymagazine.net.

Summing Up

In this chapter, we talked about adding in to fill the space that's created by all the letting go you did in the previous chapter. Some of the things you'll add in to your life include:

- Making choices every day that honor your core values

- Educating yourself about health, nutrition, and fitness

- Movement that fulfills you, works your muscles and heart, and lines up with your core values

- Healthful, nurturing foods that energize and nourish you

- Time for you to nurture yourself

- Creating a support team that can encourage you and help hold you accountable in ways that feel right for you

- Thinking about the importance of appreciation in a balanced life and brainstorming ways to pay attention to what really deserves your appreciation

In Chapter 6 we'll discuss some fantastic navigation tools and strategies that will help you stay the course as you follow a journey toward a balanced, happy life.

Chapter Six

N is for
Navigate and *Notice Nature*

I'm not afraid of storms,
for I'm learning how to sail my ship.

—Louisa May Alcott

When I was a little girl, my parents bought their first house. The inside of the house was an absolute disaster, but the minute my mother saw the backyard and the playhouse, she envisioned a beautiful home where my brother and I could run and play. The vision was so clear in her mind that she convinced my dad to buy the house, even though they had never renovated anything before.

When they moved in, my mother used her vision of the house as a guide every day, and with a very small budget, she and my father created the home of their dreams. They hit roadblocks along the way, of course—they even stripped fifteen different covers off of the countertop only to realize the counters were in horrible condition and needed to be completely replaced anyway. But they navigated their way through the challenges and achieved their goal. We lived in that house for almost two decades.

If my mother had let fear cloud out her vision, she and my dad would not have purchased the home that brought us so many amazing memories. And if they hadn't worked so hard, it would not have become the place she envisioned it could be.

Like my parents, we all face challenges as we navigate our way through life. When we have a vision for our life, we sometimes push it aside because we don't know how to make it happen. We may get frustrated with trying and choose to simply give up. I've seen this time and time again, and I've experienced it myself. But you can learn how to find your way and follow your vision without giving up on yourself.

In this chapter, we'll look at the next step of the B.A.L.A.N.C.E. Program: navigating. During this part of the program, I'll show you how to use your vision to release fear, to move forward even when you don't know exactly where you're going, to commit to your vision by taking action, and to negotiate detours along the way.

I'll also share some very effective navigational tools. First we'll talk about **mini-goal setting** and several fantastic ways to set the small, specific, everyday mini-goals that lead to real change. Next we'll look at the importance of choosing **motivators** that are **truly motivating and not energy draining.** I'll also tell you the importance of **defining your success** in ways that are healthy, realistic, and inspiring. Finally, I'll share some thoughts and tips about the wonderful value of noticing nature as you navigate through life. It's an Everyday B.A.L.A.N.C.E. Technique that is sure to bring you back to center during stressful moments.

Before we begin, I want to tell you a few things about navigating. I can absolutely help you figure out good ways for you to take inspired action in order to set and reach your goals. But I can't give you an absolute do-this, do-that blueprint. Diet books usually promise that, but it's one of the big reasons that prescribed diets fail.

Using Your Vision and Goals to Serve the World

I know you may have picked up this book because you want to lose weight. I believe you are beautiful just as you are, and I want to assist you in being the best version of yourself possible by loving yourself, getting off the dieting wheel of frustration, being an active participant in your life, and using your vision and goals to serve the world. Your life and the scale will balance out naturally!

When someone or something outside of you tries to navigate your life, failure is almost guaranteed. Only you can look within to find the steps that will allow you to successfully navigate this journey called life. And if you're setting goals, only you know yourself well enough to make a plan so customized that it will fit every part of your personality, schedule, core values, and lifestyle. But that doesn't mean you're on your own—absolutely not! Your wisdom comes from God, and He's the greatest teacher in town! And I'm with you every step of the way showing you some of the most effective tools for you and your own personal navigational system.

Sometimes women feel a little lost at this point. They want to be told exactly what to do. They want a blueprint. But let me tell you, I know from my own experience and the success of the women I've worked with that the only way to make permanent change, the only way to live a life in balance, is to look within yourself.

Once you accept that, navigating can actually be fun! Instead of being boxed in by a bunch of someone else's rules, you have the freedom to choose your own. You can do what you want to do and be who you want to be, and at the same time, you can change what you want to change.

Let me give you an example of this. One of my clients told me she had given up on exercise. She had tried everything—jogging on a treadmill, walking outdoors with friends, group exercise classes, and working with a personal trainer. None of it lit her fire. She was convinced there was no exercise that she could enjoy.

So I asked her to think about whether any of her other personal goals might give her a clue as to what kind of exercise she would like. She reviewed her personal goals and had a lightbulb moment when she thought about her goal of connecting with her husband in a more sensual way. She came up with an idea I would never have expected for her: belly dancing classes! She signed up for the classes and loved them. Belly dancing helped her reconnect with her body and appreciate its strength, which led to a greater desire to move in other ways as well. It also boosted her feelings of sensuality, which made a big difference between her and her husband. Now she's even thinking of taking a pole-dancing aerobics class!

This is such a perfect illustration of how it's so much better to look within yourself for goals and motivators than to expect some kind of one-size-fits-all plan or diet to provide them for you. It would never have occurred to me to suggest that she take up belly dancing—and honestly, even if I had suggested it, if she hadn't gone through the early steps of the B.A.L.A.N.C.E. Program, I'm sure she would have told me I was crazy. But the process of brain dumping, assessing, letting go, and adding in opened her up to listen to her inherent wisdom and discover a navigational plan that was truly her own.

You can navigate your journey by taking small inspired steps and setting mini-goals. Planning ahead of time and holding yourself accountable will help you to gain a sense of accomplishment when you put your navigation plan in motion. And if, by tapping in to your innate wisdom, you discover you really like blueprints, you will be able to create your own.

Faith and Focus

I love watching tightrope walkers at the circus—their elegance, grace, and focus inspire such awe in me. (As an aside, I always think it's odd that we use the term *three-ring circus* to describe chaos. In reality, everything done in a circus is done with precision and laser focus—it has to be, or the performers would get hurt.)

We can learn a lot about life by observing circus performers, especially the tightrope walkers. They don't focus on the fact that they are a hundred feet in the air. They don't look at all the faces staring up at them and all the circus acts going on below them, and then freeze in fear of falling. Of course not. They take just one step at a time but keep moving forward to get to the other side. They focus on the moment.

When we're doing multiple activities at once, we can't focus solely on the fact that we are doing so many things at once. This is overwhelming, and can lead to negative thoughts such as, *I am stressed—I have too much to do.* Or, *I will never get anything done.* Or, *This is impossible!*

Negativity gets you nowhere except stuck in a rut. If you have a laundry list of goals to navigate and tasks to get done and you are thinking about all of them, you can't focus on the task at hand. If you are at work and you're worrying about what to make for dinner, you'll spend more time on Google searching for twenty-minute chicken recipes than you will finishing the research you need for your presentation tomorrow. Then tomorrow morning, you'll stress about the unfinished presentation and focus more on the stress than on the task, which will lead to sloppy results.

The same is true when we are faced with a fear. I always feel far more in balance when I focus on faith instead of fear. Remember, having a positive attitude isn't just about what we say or how we present ourselves. For a positive attitude to be more than words, it must also be exemplified in our thoughts, our actions, and how we handle the situations we are presented with. It is a state of being. An attitude of faith permeates all areas of our life.

With an attitude of faith, you can have a laser focus on what you are aiming for, and then on getting it done. When you focus on the task at hand and know that something else will follow soon, you're better able to keep moving forward.

This is true for anything you want to pursue in life, even the smallest of things, like driving someplace new. If you have a map with a final destination, you take the turns one at a time. If you jump ahead to the seventh turn before you've taken the first one, you're very likely to get lost.

Try to have the same laser focus as the tightrope walker. Walk through life with grace, elegance, and faith, even when you're facing fear, chaos, or even just a long to-do list.

Knowing How to Navigate

As you are moving forward in this journey, keep this in mind: navigating should be fun! Give yourself permission to think outside the box, to consider possibilities, to try new things—you can even throw the map away sometimes. If you've been on a million diets that haven't worked, you know the standard navigational strategies won't work for you. That means you're free—you no longer have to do what the so-called diet experts recommend. You can chart your own course. Open your mind, dig deep into your soul, be guided by your personal goals and core values, and create a path that will take you where you want to go. And have fun along the way!

Don't be discouraged if your journey is slow. Creating change is like rolling a snowball. At first, the snow won't pack, and no matter how hard you try, all you have is a pile of snowflakes. But, if you stick with it, soon, *wow,* watch out world! You are rolling a snowball bigger than you ever imagined.

If you've been racking your brain thinking about how to do something you want to do or how to make a change, just do one small thing that is in line with your vision, and do it regularly. Soon the small thing will inspire you to do a little more, and a little more. If you're hungry, eat a few almonds instead of a bag of chips. Don't worry about what you'll eat tomorrow—just focus on honoring your core values and achieving small goals now.

Real change happens when the thing we want to change is practiced and made into habit. This is true with everything. Think about brushing your teeth: doing it once in a while doesn't work. You have to do it twice a day, every day, or else your teeth decay. Think about relationships: you can't go on one date a year and expect to have a meaningful relationship with someone. True love grows from a steady stream of communication and connection. Think about careers, parenting, hobbies: all are most successful when the tasks to perform each are done regularly, consistently, and with passion.

Mini-Goals:
Setting One Small Goal at a Time

Setting mini-goals is an incredibly powerful process. Even the tiniest step or action, even if it's imperfect, will move you forward in some way. When you choose daily and weekly goals, you create a clear, detailed road map that you can follow in your journey toward creating a balanced life and being the person you were meant to be. Your mini-goals tell you when to turn left, when to turn right, when to speed up, and when to slow down. And, if you make a wrong turn with a mini-goal, it's no big deal. It's just a miniature wrong turn, and you can easily get back on course.

Choosing mini-goals is an individualized process that must be based on your own personality and lifestyle. Your mini-goals reflect who you are and are different for everyone. For example, some women like very structured goals; others prefer open-ended goals. Some women write their goals down; others keep them in their heads. However, I always say give your thoughts power by putting them in motion—either by writing them down, speaking them aloud, or (this one is a must) taking inspired action. None of these strategies is best for everyone—you have to figure out what works best for you.

You may be wondering at this point how you know what mini-goals to set and what the heck inspired action means. Many women are used to a book telling them the goals they should go for. But I believe you have the answers within you. I find it quite amazing to watch women take the leap to trust themselves, be still and listen when they don't quite know the answers, and let their vision be their guide. Inspired action comes from listening. Spending quiet time to visualize and hear your inner guide helps navigation run smoothly.

Inspired action doesn't feel forced. It might not be simple and you may have to push yourself to do it, but it's coming from a deeper place within you. And even when something throws you off, you still choose to take the action.

In a workshop last month, I asked the ladies to begin navigating by setting mini-goals or intentions for the week. Penny sent the following email to the group:

> *Lying in bed last night, I made the intention that I'd get up at dawn to go for a walk in Roosevelt Park—a nice brisk walk from the parking lot by Grandview Avenue to the lake, around it, and back. It was a very good intention with a goal of getting my exercise in before sitting down at my computer.*
>
> *The alarm rang at five thirty, but I was so snuggly in bed. So I just lay there. I thought again about intentions and goals. I considered the pros and cons of staying in bed, warm, safe and*

snug, with nice quiet time to think about my goals and inten-
tions versus getting up and facing the cruel, chilly world. The
bed won, and I fell asleep! It was one of those delicious, deep
early morning sleeps—the kind you wake from naturally, all
refreshed.

I did go to Roosevelt Park, but not until nine thirty!

There is some good to this delayed intention, though. I talked
to the contractor in charge of installing the new Health Trail in
the park. He said it will be ready for use soon. It is a series of
stations where you do a few reps of an exercise—push-ups, pull-
ups, kicks, sit-ups, and so on. Then you jog or walk to the next
station. Sounds challenging and fun. My intention is to do this
on my "off" Curves day.

So here is my intention:

> *Monday, Wednesday, and Friday: Curves*
>
> *Tuesday, Thursday, and Saturday: Health Trail*
>
> *Sunday: Sleep late (or later!)*

All this boils down to a goal of being fit and trim by the end of
the summer.

As her intention shows, Penny had to push herself—her plan didn't
go exactly as she thought it would. But she was inspired by her intention and took action, and it turned out even better than she imagined.
If Penny hadn't set an intention for herself, she may have never even
considered going to the park at all.

Ask these questions to begin your navigation:

- What is my intention for today? For this week?

- How can I nurture my body, soul, and spirit?

- What step will I take today to move myself forward?

    - Will I walk around my block one time?

— Will I write a letter to an old friend I have been thinking about?

— Will I read that book that's collecting dust on the shelf?

— Will I write a grocery shopping list and stock up on energizing foods?

— Will I eat more fresh vegetables, enlist a support team, or begin strength training?

Just do one thing and get that snowball rolling. You'll soon see how exciting it is to create change just by taking a single step!

By the Numbers

Some people write the date in numbers: 8/20/10. I like to spell it out: August 20, 2010. I don't know why, but there's something about numbers that drives me a little bonkers. Of course, they are a way of quantifying things, and they are probably more tangible for some people than words are. For example, many people define success by numbers: what a job pays, what's in their bank account, what the scale says, how many bedrooms are in their home, how many hours they worked in a day. I just don't define success that way.

Success to me is living with passion, energy, and purpose. Success to me is making sure I've kissed my husband goodnight every night, even on those nights when we're affected by the Mars-Venus thing. Success to me is tickling my daughter, teaching her to write, or making my son giggle by dancing around the room with him. Success is being able to do a job I love and still have peace of mind to pay my bills and have some fun. And if money's a little tight, success is figuring out how to budget better, knowing what's important, and booking different types of work so it will be easier. Heck, some days, success is even just getting a shower, lip gloss, and matching socks on before leaving the house!

I understand that quantifying success makes it simpler for some people to measure themselves, but I think it makes it harder to figure out how to get where you want to be. I mean, sure, we can say, "I resolve to lose ten pounds," or "I want to make a six-figure salary," or "I want to be married only once." Hmmm . . . all good numbers. And, I understand, I used to also look at the end result—what I wanted in a numbers way. But, not being a numbers person, I always struggled with that perspective and was frustrated by *how* to get to those numbers.

Instead, I choose to use words to define what I really want for my life. Honestly, I don't care what the scale says, but I want to have tons of energy, feel great, and keep my body strong. Living well is a tool that helps me to do that, and yes, I've managed to get the number on the scale down too. If the computer screen tells me I have X number of dollars in the bank, it doesn't really mean anything to me. But I'd like to take my kids on day trips, go on dates with my husband, save a little for the future, and give back to the world by helping others. If I have enough money—whatever the number—for that, I'm thrilled.

TAKE ACTION

QUIZ YOURSELF:
WHICH GOAL SYSTEM WORKS BEST FOR YOU?

You may have no problem setting mini-goals for yourself, breaking it down into little daily actions, and holding yourself accountable. But for many women, it is more natural to navigate their kids' schedules or a work project than it is to navigate the vision they have for their life. I understand completely! So I recommend four different strategies for navigating. You may want to give them all a try so you can see what works best for you. And to make it even simpler to pick one to begin with, I've designed this Navigation Quiz.

Take the Navigation Quiz to figure out which navigation system may work perfectly for your personality type. Then we'll explore each type of navigation system.

1. My favorite program on the computer is:

    a. Microsoft Word

    b. Microsoft Excel

    c. PaintShop Pro

    d. What's a computer?

2. My favorite television show features:

    a. Stories about real people

    b. How things are made

    c. People creating something from scratch (food, clothes, songs)

    d. I don't watch TV

3. My favorite subject in school is/was:

    a. Literature

    b. Math and/or science

    c. Arts and crafts

    d. Philosophy

4. I send birthday greetings with a:

    a. Handwritten message inside a store-bought card via snail mail

    b. Computer message, usually an e-card or typed via email

    c. Homemade birthday card created from scratch

    d. Letter or phone call

5. When I am packing for vacation, I:

    a. Go from room to room, looking around and deciding which items from each room have to be packed

    b. Print out a master packing list that I keep on my computer

    c. Sit down beforehand and write a detailed list of all the items I have to bring

    d. Just start tossing things in my suitcase—I know intuitively what I have to pack without really thinking about it

6. When planning a vacation to Italy, I would:

    a. Read a travel guide and write down a long list of places I want to see and restaurants where I want to eat

    b. Read several travel guides, use a yellow highlighter to mark sites of interest, and create a detailed itinerary for each day of the trip

    c. Read travel guides, but wait until I'm in Italy to decide where I want to go

    d. Skip the travel guides and explore whatever moves me when I step out of my hotel each day

7. My holiday shopping strategy is:

    a. Start picking things up as I browse through stores a few weeks before the holiday

    b. Order everything online and have it wrapped a month in advance

    c. Forget shopping—I create homemade gifts for friends and family

    d. I do all my shopping in one whirlwind day

8. I have an important meeting tomorrow. My strategy for figuring out what I'm going to wear is:

    a. The night before, I picture myself in the meeting and think about what would suit me best.

    b. I have several meeting outfits that I keep pressed and ready in my closet, so I grab one in the morning and get dressed.

    c. I spend twenty minutes the night before the meeting, mixing and matching various blouses, skirts, scarves, and jewelry and create a look that will fit the occasion.

    d. I glance in my closet in the morning, spend ten seconds picking something out, and get dressed without a second thought.

9.   The spice jars in my kitchen are:

    a. In a spice rack on the wall or counter

    b. In their own spice drawer, organized in alphabetical order

    c. Located throughout my kitchen, stored with the foods they go with—for example, the oregano is on the shelf with the pasta and canned tomatoes

    d. Jammed into the cabinet over my stove

10. I file my tax returns:

    a. A few weeks before April 15

    b. In January, right after I receive my tax forms

    c. Whenever I get around to it

    d. Whenever my accountant gets around to it

If the majority of your answers are A, you are a words girl. You love to read and write. You love to hear people's stories and tell your own, so consider choosing **story goals.**

If the majority of your answers are B, you are a detail-oriented analytical thinker. You love checklists and calculators, and in school science probably made your soul stir. For a smart girl like you, consider choosing **S.M.A.R.T. goals.**

If the majority of your answers are C, you are a dreamer who sees potential in yourself and others. You are creative and visual, so consider choosing goals by **visioneering.**

If the majority of your answers are D, you are a deep thinker. You love studying philosophers and looking for the deeper meaning in things, so consider choosing **intentions.**

If your answers were all over the map, read through all the goal-setting strategies and choose what feels best to you. You'll probably end up mixing and matching a bit of each to create your own goal-setting strategy.

· ·

Story Goals: Navigate Your Way to Success by Telling a Story

If you aren't quite sure what mini-goals will help you become the person you envision, you can create a story. To do this, set aside some quiet time, get comfortable, and open your journal. Let the blank page inspire you to see what your heart desires.

Write a story about yourself as you dream of being—healthier, fitter, and with greater balance in body and mind. Then begin to write about the steps you have to take to become that person. Perhaps you tell a story about yourself exercising, shopping for healthy foods, and feeling wonderful. You can break it down a bit and write about what you'll have to do each week, and then each day, to fill the gap between where you are and where you'd like to be. Let the words pour out of you. Focus also on the benefits of your story goals. How will you feel when you are healthier and fitter? What changes might you see?

Give yourself time to think about story goals every couple of days. Each time you tell yourself your own success story, you'll envision more and you'll get more specific.

Here are some examples of story goals:

Today I am excited to walk five miles on the boardwalk. I can't wait to smell the fresh ocean air, feel the light morning breeze in my hair, and be warmed by the sun on my skin. Later, I will snuggle up on the couch and do some reading—this is a luxury I don't often give to myself!

I am in the mood to do a thorough cleaning of my office today, including the windows and desktops. My boss has been away, and I want it to look and smell nice when she returns next week. After work, I am going to the gym to do the elliptical trainer. I want to push myself, sweat, get my heart rate up, and feel my body working hard.

I know it's important to communicate better with my husband. I think today I will treat him the way I want to be treated instead of holding on to anger and resentment. Maybe I will surprise him by making him lunch and putting a note inside. He may think I've gone mad, but it's worth a shot at being romantic! I am going to spend time outside after everyone leaves—I think I will go for a long, brisk walk. Perhaps I'll even run a bit. The housework has been piling up too. I want to do the dishes, wash two loads of laundry, and dust everywhere.

Be Smart with S.M.A.R.T. Goals

S.M.A.R.T. goals are commonly used by authors, trainers, employers, and coaches. S.M.A.R.T. goal-setting is a proven, effective method for setting and accomplishing your goals. It is usually favored by people who like structure, although I've also seen some very freewheeling women warm up to S.M.A.R.T. goals. To use this process, keep these S.M.A.R.T. steps in mind as you create your mini-goals.

S is for Specific: Make your goals as specific as possible because specific goals are much more effective than general goals. They allow you to zero in on exactly what you want to achieve. For example, a general goal may be to exercise. A specific goal is detailed, targeted, and fully described: to walk for thirty minutes on the high school track five mornings a week at an intensity that elevates your heart rate to your target zone. Specific goals offer you a clear picture and an unambiguous story line that is easy to follow.

M is for Measurable: Be sure to establish concrete ways to track and measure your progress. For example, if your goal is to walk five days a week, use a calendar, chart, or spreadsheet to keep track of how frequently you walk, how long or far you go, and other details. This will give you a very clear sense of your progress and achievement, and you'll be able to easily track whether you've reached your targeted goals each day, week, month, quarter, and so on. When you meet your mini-goals, you'll see and feel your positive results in a way that inspires you to continue to work hard to live the healthy life you envision.

To make sure your goal is measurable, ask yourself questions such as: How long? How many? How much? How will I know when my goal is accomplished? Set realistic measurement periods—for example, keep a weekly walking log and evaluate your success every Sunday night. If you meet your goal, congratulate yourself, spend a few minutes celebrating your dedication and enjoying how it feels to succeed, and then channel that positive energy into your next week's goal.

A is for Attainable: Set realistic, attainable goals that you can actually achieve. Unattainable goals are impossible to achieve and only cause frustration and negativity. For example, if you decide you'll lose ten pounds in one weekend, not only will you fail to reach your goal, but you'll also feel bad for having failed. But if you set an attainable goal, one that is truly in your power to achieve, you are in complete control. If you want to achieve it, you can. An example of an attainable goal is to start your weekend with a fifteen-mile bike ride and to eat at least five fruits and vegetables each day.

That's not to say you should set the bar so low you can't possibly fail. If you make goals *too* attainable, you won't feel excited and energized when you achieve them. Having lofty goals is a great idea—I firmly believe that just about anything is possible to a willing heart. But the best way to achieve a hard-to-reach goal is to break it up into smaller, attainable steps. If you've never run more than a mile and you decide you want to run a marathon, good for you! But don't expect to go from sedentary to athletic in one week. Instead, set a series of attainable mini-goals that will allow you to move at a steady pace toward achieving your larger goal.

If you commit to your vision, believe in yourself, and do the work, you can figure out the steps to make it happen. Think about the abilities, skills, resources, and attitude you need to create changes. You'll be amazed at yourself when a goal that once seemed out of reach has become your reality because you've stretched yourself.

R is for Relevant: Your goals have to be relevant and must mesh with your personality, your current state of mind, and the realities of your lifestyle. If you're a night owl, planning to get up at five A.M. every day to go to the gym is a goal that's destined to fail because it doesn't align with who you are. Set goals that take your life's realities into account.

T is for Tangible: A goal is tangible when you can see it, feel it, touch it, or count it. It is something real you can work toward, not simply an idea. There is less room for subjectivity when a goal is tangible. For example, setting a goal to raise funds for an event is far different from setting a goal to enlist five people to each raise $200 in thirty days. They can accomplish their goal by selling twenty tickets each, less than one ticket per day.

S.M.A.R.T. goals should answer the six *W* questions.

Who: Who is involved?

What: What do I want to create?

Why: Why is this important to me? What are the benefits?

When: Set your time frame. Hold yourself accountable.

Where: Establish a location.

Which: Identify your obstacles and strategize to overcome them.

I have worked with some women who create three S.M.A.R.T. goals per week and others who create one or two daily. Choose what feels best for you. You may find that writing out your S.M.A.R.T. goals on Sunday sets you up nicely for the week ahead, or you may realize that writing your goal daily with your morning coffee revs you up for the day!

Here are some examples of S.M.A.R.T. goals:

Weekly: Between Monday and Friday, in order to strengthen muscles, I will do three sets of eighteen repetitions per muscle group with Nautilus equipment at the gym. I will break it up into three strength-training workouts on Monday (upper body), Wednesday (lower body), and Friday (midsection) at four thirty P.M.

Daily: I will elevate my heart rate to 70 to 80 percent during my Curves workout at noon today.

Weekly: I will eat three fresh fruits daily and four fresh vegetables daily. I will drink sixty-four ounces of water with lemon each day. I will call my best friend and spend at least thirty minutes on the phone with her so we can catch up. I will write and mail thank-you notes to everyone who came to my birthday party.

Create Your Vision by Visioneering

The key to realizing a dream is to focus not on success
but significance—and then even the small steps and little
victories along your path will take on greater meaning.

—Oprah Winfrey

We've already discussed the importance of having a vision that is connected to you in a profound, meaningful way. In Chapter 2, you spent some time crafting a vision statement and a vision board. You may have even expanded upon your vision while reading the subsequent chapters. You can use your vision as a daily guide, looking to your vision for inspired action steps that will move you forward in creating it. I call this visioneering.

I love the visioneering method because it taps in to our innate power as human beings to literally create what we imagine. Visioneering is deeper than just having the vision itself. More specifically, it is made up of four distinct components: vision, knowing, listening, and taking inspired action.

Go back to the vision of your life you created while brain dumping in Chapter 2. Then try the following steps.

1. **Schedule time to visualize.** To some of us, visualization comes naturally. That's how it is with me. Visions appear when I wake up, in moments throughout the day, and before I go to bed at night. But that doesn't happen for everyone. When you're consumed by a packed schedule or repressed by the practical voice of a loved one, visualization can seem a little frivolous, almost like daydreaming. But trust me, it is far beyond daydreaming. A daydream is picturing yourself on a secluded island sipping a piña colada. Visualizing taps in to your core being, who you were born to be, and your best self

using your gifts and your talents, feeling awakened and alive right where you are on the grass that's beneath your feet in this moment. Waking yourself up to your vision gives you the permission to open your internal floodgates and let the vision out of hiding.

So if visualizing doesn't happen in a natural way for you, schedule the time to do it—when you wake up, at lunch, before you go to sleep. If you don't plan it, it may not happen. Start simply, with five minutes. After a while you'll start doing it naturally and automatically. Again, there really are no rules—you can close your eyes and think about your vision, write in your journal, or create a collage of pictures or a scrapbook. Pin pictures and notes to cork board in your bedroom or office; slip clippings and pictures into a photo box; or file goals, visions, and pictures neatly in an organizer. One of my clients has a vision wall in her bedroom. She hangs quotes, pictures, words, drawings, and even textures there. She felt she was too hard on people, so she used a piece of soft, velvet fabric as the backdrop for her wall to represent the fact that in her balanced life vision, she is softer with people. Do whatever makes your vision come alive for you.

2. **Make it breathe with your knowing.** A vision becomes more alive when you have a *knowing* around it. We not only hope and believe it will come to be, we *know* it will. It's in our hearts, it's in our being. Because of so many yo-yo diets, you may not really believe you can lose weight. But if you fully commit and believe in yourself, you'll begin to know that you'll succeed. Remember, you are not trying to make your vision happen. You are simply being who you were born to be. Connect with your vision and commit to it.

Listen to your inner critic for a moment, and then tell her to take a hike. Notify your inner critic that she is no longer allowed to take up space in your brain. Don't repress her or sweep her under the rug. You are dumping her, kicking her to the curb! When that inner critic voice takes you away from the state of knowing, it's like sticking a pin in a balloon. The vision loses its air, its power. Try to have a knowing with yourself the same way you would believe in your best friend. If your best friend was saying she was a failure, she was doubtful, she was unsure of her gifts in this world, you would probably go bananas telling her how crazy she sounded. Use your own internal knowing to do the same for yourself.

3. **Listen to your heart.** Listening is very powerful and often underestimated. I know sometimes we have a vision that we want so badly to make happen, that we go like gangbusters to succeed. But you can't bully a vision and ram it into action. Vision flows gracefully, and the steps should be somewhat intuitive. How does a visioneer know what steps to take? Often just by listening. When you stop and listen—really listen— you open yourself to hearing something deeper that you may not have heard when you were running around like a maniac. Stillness is an action that gives voice to your inner wisdom.

   I know you don't live in a bubble. And I completely understand that quieting your mind is much more easily said than done. But it gets easier with practice. Quiet your inner critic, breathe deeply, perhaps close your eyes and picture something serene, such as a white light, a blank canvas, or still water— and then just listen.

4. **Take inspired action.** You have created your vision, silenced your inner critic, and taken a moment to listen. You have a clear picture of the way you want to feel, look, communicate, breathe, be. Knowing all that, you can align your actions with your goals and take action inspired by your vision. By being what you see in your mind's eye, you fulfill your vision in a natural, organic way.

   Throughout the day, stop and ask yourself if what you are

about to do is in line with your vision of being balanced and healthy: Going for a walk? Yes, it is. Being stagnant all day? No, it isn't. Speaking kind words and being compassionate? Yes, it is. Yelling and getting frustrated at every turn? No, it isn't.

Visioneering is engineering your vision as you mindfully maneuver and navigate through life. Taking these four steps will help move the vision into your reality!

Change by Making an Intention

An intention is a powerful energy that we often don't realize we are using. Intention can direct your mind in an aware, conscious way. You put your decision in motion by putting it in words, followed by taking the inspired actions that support it.

Whenever I teach workshops, I ask the participants what their intention is with taking the class. Many women respond with a simple "My intention is to lose weight." This is an outcome, not necessarily an intention, but it begins the process of living with intention.

Intention is more encompassing than the outcome, the goals, or even the objectives. Intentions are a way of being in the world. Using intention to navigate your journey is surprisingly powerful. You may begin to consciously state your intentions. And of course, they may at first seem more like goals or desires, but over time, your intentions will become clearer. One woman on our last day of class ran in the door excited to speak to me before the others arrived. She exclaimed, "I get it! I know my intention. My intention is to be in balance!" She then explained that just by knowing her intention, she felt more in balance.

Intentions do not have to be overwhelming. As a matter of fact, a simple thought or statement can carry a lot of power, sometimes more than an entire paragraph can. Here are some examples:

- Today I will be kind and nurturing to myself and others.

- This week I will be plugged in to the world around me.

- I intend to live each day fully, to be powerful in body, mind, and spirit.

Another way to make intentions is to place an intention *on* something that will help keep you focused on your goals. One woman from the workshop did this when she was going to a wedding. She knew nobody on the guest list, and she worried that she would feel socially awkward and would soothe her anxiety by spending the evening eating. I suggested that when she entered the reception room, she metaphorically place an intention on something in the room that reflected one of her core values and that she could relate to in a positive way. One of her core values is elegance, so she placed an intention on the gorgeous orchid centerpiece on her table. Throughout the evening, whenever she felt socially awkward or tempted to overeat, she looked at the orchid centerpiece and reminded herself that she could handle social situations with grace and elegance. The centerpiece was a talisman of sorts—something that could remind her of her intention whenever she needed a bit of support and encouragement. It worked like a charm, so to speak—she got through the reception without overeating or feeling completely out of place.

Which navigation strategies should you use? Go with your gut. They should feel comfortable, and even if at first you have to work at navigating, once you begin, it should become a natural part of you.

Choose Motivation That Really Motivates

A few years ago, a woman told me she had a great technique for losing weight. She hung a big sign above her scale that said, "How will I lose the last ten pounds?"

She weighed herself daily, sometimes even more than once a day, and the sign was meant to motivate her to lose more weight. I was curious about her method, so naturally I inquired more about it. She then went on to tell me, while the sign was meant to motivate her, she could not answer the question of how. She knew what she wanted to do, but she didn't know how—and that was a huge source of frustration for her. And that's what led her to me.

For her, using S.M.A.R.T. goals took away the frustration. She is a numbers person—she set goals to walk a certain number of minutes, reach a certain heart rate, and eat a certain number of fruits and vegetables. Those numbers were perfect action steps for her, and they helped her finally lose those last ten pounds. But if you're not a numbers person, that would be energy draining.

Motivating behavior propels you to make change. If visioneering doesn't help you change, it's not motivating. I met a woman who tried to motivate herself by hanging up a picture of herself as a slim, trim high school student. She looked to the photo for inspiration and motivation, but week after week, she couldn't change her behavior. When I asked her about it, she realized the problem: "Every time I look at it, I feel disgusted with myself." I told her to throw the picture away because it wasn't motivating change—it was draining her energy! This method might work for some people, but it clearly wasn't working for her.

The best way to motivate yourself is to figure out what kind of motivation works well for you. Again, this is very personal; what motivates me might drive you crazy, and vice versa. You have to tap in to what you already know about yourself. Here are some questions to ask yourself to help you determine what motivates you:

- What motivates me in other parts of my life where I am a success?

- What am I good at?

- What do I enjoy?

- What drives me?

- What do I thrive on?

Here are some motivators that the women I've worked with have shared with me:

- Having someone to hold you accountable

- Checking off boxes on a chart

- Rewards

- Deadlines

- Trying on clothing

- The energetic feeling you get from exercising

- The effect your positive change has on other people

Once you figure out what your positive motivators are, make the most of them. If you enjoy the praise and encouragement of others, join or form a support group. If you love numbers, use charts and check boxes that measure your success. If you're visually oriented, use color and pictures or graphic software to create charts and graphs. Take a look at what you're doing in the name of motivation. If the behavior is accelerating change in a positive, healthy way, that's fantastic. But if it's causing you stress or frustration, it's time to make a change!

Be Flexible When the Winds Change

When I was in high school, my family decided to take a road trip to South Carolina. My father is very reminiscent of Chevy Chase in the *Vacation* movies—he was super-excited, planned every detail, and had itineraries and road stops all mapped out ahead of time. What he didn't figure into his calculations was the fact that my mother, siblings, and I would all fall asleep during the ride, so he didn't have anyone to help navigate.

A couple of missed turns, and we were in the car for an extra couple hours. Now, I'm sure he wasn't the happiest when he was trying to figure out how to get us back on course, but we ended up near a unique place called South of the Border. In my father's original mapped-out plan, we would have missed it. As it turned out, our family had an absolute blast at the place that we may have never gone to if his plan had worked perfectly.

We are all a bit like Chevy Chase (and my father) as we plan our life journey. We pick a destination and head straight for it. But sometimes we get lost and the best, unexpected things happen. When we're blown off course, we learn lessons, we connect more with each other and with nature, and we often find happiness.

It's great to have a vision—knowing where we want to go and taking the steps we need to get there. But the next time your road map takes you on a detour, trust in the absolute power that life has a beautiful way of unfolding perfectly as it should.

Everyday B.A.L.A.N.C.E. Technique:
Notice Nature

As you know, my Everyday B.A.L.A.N.C.E. Techniques are designed as a way to find balance during stressful moments. You've learned to stop to breathe, accept, laugh, and appreciate. Now it's time to notice nature. It's easy to get wrapped up in the hustle and bustle of life, but if you are in a bit of a funk or feeling stressed out to the max, take notice of the nature that surrounds you. You are bound to lower your blood pressure, calm your body, appreciate more, and even learn a lesson or two.

And what you notice in nature actually holds a mirror up to what is within you already. Twenty people may look at the same view and each see something completely different. You can discover much about yourself just by looking at the world around you. Not only is it sooth-ing to watch a bird fly, to smell a flower, to stare at a starry sky, but it is also a way to learn a bit about ourselves.

Sitting on my front porch is one of the great joys of my life. Today I focused on all the beautiful foliage right across from our home. We don't live in a secluded area—in fact, the highway is just a few turns away. And yet, there is so much natural beauty right outside my door.

As I enjoyed the leaves, this quote popped into my mind:

Adopt the pace of nature; her secret is patience.

—Ralph Waldo Emerson

I can't even imagine how old they are, how many stories they have to tell, the sage trees that surround our home. Nature is patient.

There are many things in my life that I want to unfold, and I'm sure the same is true for you. You may remember Veruca's famous line from *Willy Wonka and the Chocolate Factory,* "I want it *now!*" We may not stomp our feet, but I think we all feel like Veruca some-times, especially when we have our minds made up about something. But patience is a virtue. We shouldn't wait in anticipation for life to happen. It happens naturally as it should, moment to moment. And, as Emerson points out, we must adopt the pace of nature.

Today it dawned on me that the trees are all imperfectly gorgeous and unique. Nature is beautiful, but not perfect. The trees don't line up standing the same height wearing the same shade of brown. They are scattered, their branches varying in size, shape, and color. They are chipped, worn, and spotted. Nature is flawed perfectly.

There are so many lessons right before our eyes if we just open them and take a look around. Today, think of something you've been wanting, anticipating, and let it go. Let go of the need for perfection. Trust everything will all work out in time, and enjoy each moment.

TAKE ACTION

RUN A RAINY-DAY MILK BATH

LuLu, Little Man, and I often go to our front porch when it rains. We love just watching the rain fall. The kids are calmer on the porch when it rains—it relaxes their energetic little bodies. And it is such a wonder to witness the drops covering the blades of grass and Lu's flower petals in uniquely beautiful patterns; the sound is soothing to our ears.

I think rain gets a bad rap. Sure, it may cause delays when you're traveling or create frizz in a freshly blown-out head of hair, but I think it is nature's way of telling us to stop and breathe. It's fun to embrace the rain, and when it's a soft rain, I like to relax right along with it. Sometimes a rainstorm inspires me to take a milk bath using a simple homemade mix that has healing benefits to the body.

Makes 1 bath.

What You'll Need

2 cups whole milk

1 cup sea salt

1 cup baking soda

Let's Do This

In a large bowl, mix together the milk, sea salt, and baking soda. Run your bath to a warm temperature, and pour the mixture in. Set a serene mood by lighting candles and turning off the light switch. Leave the books on the bookshelf and turn your mind off. Open your windows, let the breeze flow through, and just listen to the rain.

Milk has natural softening and soothing properties. (Cleopatra knew this—she took frequent milk baths to keep her skin fresh and beautiful.) Milk contains lipids that deeply moisturize the skin. Sea salt helps improve circulation, assists in rejuvenating the cells, and completely relaxes the body. Baking soda is known as a detoxifier that helps you feel re-energized and has an alkalizing effect that counters the acidity typically caused by red meats, cheese, sugar, and refined foods. All those benefits, plus soft skin and relaxation too!

. . . .

Summing Up

In this chapter, we talked about the following navigation strategies:

- How to use your vision of a balanced life to navigate your way through challenges and obstacles

- The importance of setting mini-goals

- Four fabulous goal-setting strategies that can guide you in customizing goals to your personality, schedule, and way of looking at life: story goals, S.M.A.R.T. goals, visioneering, and intentions

- Ways to find motivators that energize rather than drain energy

In Chapter 7, we'll determine what specific obstacles may get in the way of achieving your goals, identify surefire ways to confront them, and formulate a plan that you can use to set out clear, specific ways to hold yourself accountable to your goals and vision.

. . . .

Chapter Seven

C is for
Confront and *Connect*

Life's challenges are not supposed
to paralyze you; they're supposed to
help you discover who you are.

—Bernice Johnson Reagon

. . . .

When I was little, I loved bowling. My parents began taking me to the lanes as soon as I was old enough to stand, and they let me have a go at it. Back then there were no bumpers in the gutters, but it didn't matter. The fact that I got to roll the ball made me happy, and even if no pins fell, I would jump up and down and make a happy fuss.

As I moved from bowling for fun into a kids' league, I started to take it more seriously, and I only wanted to get strikes or spares. Of course, I would miss sometimes, and it would really make me mad. Instead of a happy fuss, I made a mad one.

I'll never forget my father's words after one of my meltdowns when I said I was giving up the sport. I was sick of not being able to break 100.

"Jennie, great bowlers become great bowlers because they love the game. They hone their skills, they get gutter balls, and they learn from their mistakes. They mess up, but they never give up."

That lesson has stuck with me in many ways throughout my life, and I think of it whenever something doesn't go as planned. Love the journey. Keep working, learning, experiencing, and most importantly, keep going.

Life is full of obstacles and challenges. You hit a traffic jam on the way home from work. You plan to make a salad for dinner and realize you're out of lettuce. As you run out the door to an exercise class, your daughter unexpectedly asks for a ride to her friend's house. Life throws plenty of big obstacles at you too—job layoffs, health problems, the end of a marriage, the loss of a loved one. And then there are the obstacles that come from deep inside you—fear, self-doubt, despair, resignation. All these obstacles can throw you off balance and distract you from fulfilling your goals and your life vision.

Obstacles are an inevitable, unavoidable part of life. But that doesn't mean you are powerless when they occur. In fact, if you put yourself in the right frame of mind, you actually have way more power than you realize to cope with all kinds of challenges. You truly do have power within you to confront life's obstacles and stay in balance—or if they knock you off your feet, you have the power to pick yourself up and begin again on your journey of living a happy, healthy life.

In this step of the B.A.L.A.N.C.E. Program, we'll talk about how to confront your challenges, harness your inner power, and prevent obstacles from throwing you off balance on the scale and in life.

First, we'll work on defining the obstacles that prevent you from meeting your goals. To do this, we'll use some terrific tools, including the **energy sappers exercise,** which will assist you in identifying what is depleting your energy—including life's **incompletes and tolerations.** Finally, I'll give you tips on how to **surmount your obstacles** by confronting the source of your roadblocks head-on.

At the end of the chapter, I'll explain the value of **connecting,** an

Everyday B.A.L.A.N.C.E. Technique that will help you find strength from others as you face all of life's obstacles.

Identifying Your Everyday Obstacles

A few years back, I had a meeting scheduled with a woman named Cindy. Our appointment was set for 9:00 A.M. When she showed up at 9:07 A.M., frazzled by her lateness, she proceeded to spend eight minutes explaining why she was late: although she had started the morning on schedule, it took her a bit longer than she had expected to get ready, get the kids up, make lunches, feed the dog, wait for the school bus, and sit in morning traffic. So our appointment actually began at 9:15 A.M.

Cindy knew she was cutting it tight, but she figured that *somehow* her superwoman ways would get her to my office on time. Instead, the original seven-minute delay snowballed throughout her overscheduled day. By the time dinnertime rolled around, Cindy was running so late that she had to grab takeout for dinner instead of making the stir-fry she'd planned.

So many of the women I meet are like Cindy. Their day is filled with back-to-back commitments and a to-do list that doesn't stop. Some even tell me that they wish they didn't have to sleep so they'd have more time to get things done! I understand—our lives are busy. But if your day is jam-packed, self-care falls by the wayside and finding balance is just about impossible.

Confronting Serious Problems

If you are struggling with deep-seated emotional issues such as uncontrolled eating disorders, major relationship conflicts, trauma, abuse, unresolved grief, clinical depression, or other mental health problems, you probably need more help than a book can give you. If so, please seek help from a psychologist, therapist, grief counselor, or other mental health care provider. These trained professionals can help you confront painful issues in a safe, constructive way.

For Cindy, being unrealistic about how much time she needed for the tasks on her daily calendar was an obstacle that plagued her on an everyday basis. Five minutes here and eight minutes there added up throughout the day, leaving her with no time in the evening to prepare a healthy dinner, exercise, take care of herself, relax, enjoy time with her family, and get to bed on time.

Once Cindy understood and acknowledged this, she began giving herself more time for her daily tasks. Immediately she started to feel less stressed and more focused. She stopped having to waste time explaining her lateness, and instead of feeling frantic at the end of the day, she had energy left for herself.

TAKE ACTION

WHAT'S STANDING IN YOUR WAY?

You can't confront your obstacles if you don't know what they are. So take some time to identify what's getting in your way on your journey toward balance. Spend a few minutes at the end of each day looking at the goals you set for the day and tracking whether you achieved them. Then ask yourself about the goals you didn't meet. What got in the way? Were your goals realistic? Did you schedule enough time to do the tasks on your list? What (or who) interfered with your ability to do what you planned to do?

Write your daily barriers and obstacles in your B.A.L.A.N.C.E. Journal for a week or two. Then go back and look for trends. Does one particular obstacle keep popping up? Does the same problem get in your way day after day? Analyze why these things keep happening. Are you saying yes when you should be saying no? Are you being unrealistic about your schedule, about how much time you have, and about how much time tasks take? Are you keeping your schedule in your head instead of writing it down in a reliable planner?

Obstacles are the rule, not the exception! Everyone has them.

I find that there are four everyday obstacles that most commonly interfere with finding balance in life and on the scale. There are many more, and all of these four present themselves in dozens of ways. But overall, these are the biggest roadblocks for most women:

1. Overscheduling and overcommitting to activities

2. Lack of communication at home and in the workplace

3. Becoming so preoccupied with the little things in life that you don't have time or energy to think about the bigger picture

4. Under-prioritizing yourself and the gift of life

Once you identify your obstacles, you can figure out what to do to get back on track. Do you need a new scheduling system? Should you plan to exercise in the morning when you feel energized rather than in the evening when you usually feel too tired to get moving? Should you watch less television so you have more time to prepare healthy meals?

As you analyze your everyday obstacles and brainstorm solutions, start making changes in your daily goals. Continue to keep track of what you achieve and what you don't, and make specific plans for what to do when certain obstacles arise. Soon you'll start to have much more control over your everyday obstacles.

. . . .

A great way to turn everyday obstacles into opportunities for change is to create your ideal schedule. This is a fun activity, and very helpful! On a blank calendar, fill in your ideal schedule. Create it without limitations or obstacles. (But be realistic—you can't just go to the spa all day.) Remember to factor in your life vision, your day design, and your core values. Think about the gift of each day and how you would like to spend it.

If you have children, remember time is a gift to them too. If they are scheduled to the hilt with activities, they aren't able to appreciate sitting around the table having a family dinner, lying in the grass, or playing old-fashioned board games like Monopoly or Trivial Pursuit.

Designing your ideal schedule will allow you to include activities you want to do but think you don't have time for, and it may very well lead to transforming what feels like a daydream into a reality. This happened with Sandy, who said she wanted to do more volunteer work. She loved volunteering, but months and sometimes years would go by without her doing any volunteer work. She was so busy with her kids and work and everything in between that she couldn't find time. She also thought it would be good to get her kids involved in some volunteer activities.

In Sandy's ideal schedule, her kids' after-school and evening activities were limited to Mondays and Wednesdays. That would leave Tuesday and Thursday evenings open, giving Sandy and her children time to volunteer at the senior center or the children's hospital. Her ideal schedule also made room for her and her family to prepare a home-cooked meal at least one night a week. And it included time for her to go to the gym and to relax with her friends. Sandy's ideal schedule was much different from her real life, but by simply going through the exercise of imagining an ideal schedule, Sandy became excited about taking better control of her life.

Over the next few months, Sandy consciously thought of her ideal schedule and how she could change her family's current schedule accordingly. She spoke with her husband about her desire to hit the gym early in the morning, and he was all for it! He knew she felt better when she exercised. As it came time to enroll/re-enroll her kids in activities, Sandy helped her children decide which were most important and which could be dropped. With fewer activities, Sandy found time at least twice a month to volunteer, either by herself or with her kids or husband.

Another way to confront your everyday obstacles is to change the way you communicate about your time. If you need to change the way you value and use time, be sure to share this information with the people in your life so they can understand and honor your needs.

The way you value your time often reflects the way you value yourself. And the way you value yourself often is reflected back in the way others value you. This often isn't conscious, and many people don't even realize they are doing it—it just happens organically among us.

When we share and communicate openly, we change the energy of our relationships, and we change the energy we carry within ourselves, which in turn creates a more confident self.

In order to reflect a different message about yourself and your time, you must be clear about what you want. Before opening up discussion with others, write about it in your B.A.L.A.N.C.E. Journal. Let's say you are working more than you want, and it's affecting your relationship with your family and yourself. You want to tell your coworkers that you need a break. Write out what you want from the situation:

> *I am exhausted. I work day and night, and it never feels good enough. I feel like a pancake spread too thin. I have no time for me, no time with my family, and you constantly e-mail or call even after I've left work. I just want some time to relax and be with my kids and my husband. Can you please give me some space? You are overbearing, and you expect way too much from me as an employee.*

Read it back as if you were the recipient of the information, and hear it as though someone is telling it to you. Does it sound harsh? Are you immediately on the defensive? If so, reframe it in a positive, productive way. There's probably some great information in there that may be clouded by insults or venting.

Remember, the goal of communicating effectively is not to belittle or to blow up. The goal is to change the way the recipient views and values your time. If an overbearing boss doesn't let you sleep at night because your BlackBerry is ding-ding-dinging, remember you taught him that it was okay to do that by answering the call, even if you only answered once. Be honest, acknowledge the positive, acknowledge your part in the miscommunication, and then state what you are choosing. According to licensed psychotherapist and relationship expert Dr. Tom Kersting, the way in which a message is delivered to the recipient (in this case, your boss) is perhaps more important than the message itself. Dr. Tom told me, "The majority of folks, including bosses, are defensive by nature, so the delivery of your message must strike a positive chord with your recipient so that the walls of defensiveness do not emerge." He even shared a script with a better way to communicate your message:

> *I have been thinking about my wonderful life over the past few weeks, and although I appreciate all that I've been blessed with, I am exhausted. I feel like a pancake spread too thin. I love my job so much that I find myself continuing to work from home in the evenings when I should be unwinding, reading to the kids, and spending quality time with my spouse.*
>
> *I know that I'm always quick to respond to my BlackBerry, and that is my fault. My engrossment in work has taken its toll on my family, and on me, so I've decided that I need to dedicate my time after work exclusively to my family. Doing so is not only right, it gives me fulfillment, and the more fulfilled I am, the more productive I can be at work. From now on, I am going to turn my BlackBerry off after work, my kids are going to turn off the television, my husband is going to turn off the computer, and we are going to spend time together the way a family should.*

Your Circles of Life

We tend to compartmentalize our lives into separate areas. Family is in one bucket, career is in another, health is in another, and so on. But that's not how it is in real life. If you're worried about your career, it impacts your relationships. If you're constantly butting heads with your teenage son, it affects your ability to nurture your creative side. When any one of these life areas is out of balance, it drains energy from all the others—and it gets in the way of a self-care plan that includes exercising, eating a healthy diet, and losing weight.

It's not easy to put your finger on the root issues you are facing. They often have nothing to do with weight loss at all. That's why it's important to look at your whole life as you set out to identify the ob-

Zen Quickie

Silence Your Inner Drama Queen

Women waste too much of their precious time on unnecessary drama, according to Melody Stevens, master efficiency coach and creator of Time Millionaire. Give up gossiping, complaining, whining, and the drama, she advises. Doing so can give you as much as ten extra hours a week. To silence your inner drama queen, breathe a silent *om* (pronounced *aum*). Not only does this instantly relax you, but doing it daily in twenty-minute intervals can elicit what's known as the relaxation response, according to mind/body expert Herbert Benson, MD, of the Benson-Henry Institute for Mind Body Medicine at Massachusetts General Hospital. When you elicit the relaxation response, your heart beats more slowly, your blood pressure goes down, your muscles relax, and your body cuts back on the production of stress hormones such as cortisol.

stacles that trip you up. Referring back to the Balanced Inspirista graphic on page 88 can help.

We can learn so much about ourselves just by looking at the different areas of our lives, including our surroundings. I remember moving into my first apartment like it was yesterday. I walked in, laid down on the floor, and decided to paint the room orange. I was feeling happy and independent, and orange felt like a good fit.

After about six months of living on my own and going through some tricky times with relationships—listening to too much Tori Amos and developing a taste for Modigliani's artwork—I painted my orange walls deep plum. When my mother saw the room, she seemed quite concerned. "Is everything okay?" she asked.

I guess I was in a funk and didn't really see it until my mother asked me about my decor. The funk had a deeper effect on me than just the color of the walls, though. I realized that even though the scale was down, I suddenly wasn't nurturing myself. I again wasn't feeling good enough, I ate very little in fear of gaining weight, I stopped enjoying food that I loved so much, and I focused so much on food that it became my adversary. Even though years before I had learned that self-love was the key to being healthy, I suddenly wasn't being kind to myself or my body anymore. My surroundings reflected this.

Often the choices we make about our living environment, clothes, and hair reflect what we're thinking. But having deep-plum walls and mopey artwork magnified my sadness, and I lived up to my own expectation of being a woman scorned. I ate less, feared weight gain tremendously, and began avoiding full-length mirrors again. I was clearly not in balance or appreciating my body, my gifts, or my life. Even though I was in the beginning stages of helping women become healthier, I realized by my deep-plum walls that I was once again struggling to find balance.

The community of women at Curves came to my rescue. While I was trying to find my balanced self, many of our members lifted me up. Our club was decorated in a very inspirational way—phrases on the walls and encouraging words everywhere. Frenchie, a dear friend and member, noticed I wasn't myself. One day, she asked what was going on, and I released a little on her, just dumped out the dating disasters I was having. She smiled at me, a deep, loving smile, and simply pointed to the words I picked out myself that were in frames and on the walls that were chosen to inspire others. She knew I could use the encouragement and inspiration that day. Frenchie's simple concern was just what I needed.

I know that being surrounded by positive energy in the form of people, words, music, memories that make me smile, and images of dreams for my future have made all the difference in how I nurture and care for my body, how I have overcome obstacles and challenges in my life, and how I have been able to help others do the same.

You may not have changed your wall color or taken any other drastic measures, at least not that you are aware of yet. But using my

Balanced Inspirista graphic will help you define obstacles and barriers in every part of your life. Notice that surrounding the inspirista are the eight circles that make up most people's lives:

1. **Relationships:** The dynamics, effects, and growth of all personal and business relationships

2. **Physical Environment:** The space you're in at home, in your office, in your car, and elsewhere in your world

3. **Personal Development:** A clear path of development as it relates to your relationship with yourself and others

4. **Fun and Play:** Activities that support self-expression

5. **Finance:** Your concerns about money

6. **Career:** The many aspects of your work life and career path

7. **Wellness:** The various aspects of your physical, mental, emotional, and spiritual health

8. **Gifts and Creativity:** That which makes your soul stir

Remember from Chapter 2, your overall balance is made up of not only your lifestyle factors but also your internal muscle, your body, and your caring balance—so the stronger *you* are in the center of your world, the less impact each out-of-balance area may have on other areas of your life.

Remember, that while the circles of life are "surrounding" the inspirista, the circles of life still are interrelated. You are in the center. All the circles pass through you, and what happens in one circle goes through you and impacts the other circles. In my case, bad relationships impacted my physical environment, my physical environment then impacted my relationship with myself, and my relationship with myself became less than nurturing, impacting my wellness. The impact each circle has on the other varies from person to person, so you may want to create your own, noting your specific life circles and intertwining those that impact each other.

Are UHOs Throwing You Off Balance?

Unidentified hidden obstacles (UHOs) can mess with your life balance. UHOs are tricky to identify because they are the root (or source) of the challenge. The UHO is usually different from the symptom that is presenting itself to you. A symptom may be weight gain, unhappy relationships, or even lack of time. If you focus only on the symptoms, your obstacles will keep popping up like a Whac-A-Mole. But if you treat things at the root or source, you solve them for the long term. So, let's identify the UHO, so you can stop using diets to treat your symptoms.

And what's more exciting is that in most UHOs, there are extremely valuable lessons to be learned about ourselves and our lives.

You may be getting tripped up by unidentified hidden obstacles if:

- You're not meeting the goals you set

- Your tools don't seem to work

- You have trouble moving forward and creating a vision

- You aren't living up to the vision you set for yourself

- You are getting frustrated or angry with yourself

- You have trouble meeting your mini-goals

- You feel stressed by your goals

- You have a feeling that something is holding you back, but you're not sure what it is

TAKE ACTION

WHAT'S SAPPING YOUR ENERGY?

Write your life categories each on a separate page in your B.A.L.A.N.C.E. Journal. You can use the eight categories listed on page 229, or you can use your own. Find a quiet space and think about each area. Ask yourself: What is draining my energy in this life area? What is causing conflict? What worries me? What keeps me up at night? What gets on my nerves?

As you contemplate all your life categories, consider your energy sappers, including tolerations and incompletes.

Tolerations are irritants, inconveniences, aggravations, and annoyances that you barely even notice are sapping your energy. You tolerate them, either because you don't feel like dealing with them or you don't even realize they're bothering you. Some examples include a leaky faucet, the 1980s wallpaper in your dining room, the mess in your refrigerator, chronic heartburn, and the piles of junk on your basement stairs. When most women really start to think about it, they find tons of tolerations in their lives. The good news is that most tolerations can be improved or eliminated—you just have to look around, notice them, and brainstorm ways to get in control of them. Your energy will surge when you tear down that awful wallpaper and put on a fresh coat of paint, perform a kamikaze cleanup on your refrigerator, or see your doctor for advice on reducing or eliminating your heartburn. Freeing up that energy will give you more space to focus on achieving your most important goals.

Incompletes are energy sappers that result from unfinished business tugging at your mind. Examples include an insurance form that you filled in but never submitted, an overdue mammogram, a friend you no longer speak to but think about often, and a thank-you note that's three months overdue. As with tolerations, you can stop the energy drain that incompletes cause by identifying them and brainstorming ways to complete them so you can then push them out of your mind.

During my search for balance, I began taking classes to understand it better. What I learned validated my own experience, and I was now given some tools so I could help people better. I learned about the importance of looking at your whole life, your energy sappers, and your incompletes and tolerations from Stephen Cluney, a master coach and teacher at New York University. This has had a profound effect on me personally, and on many of the women I worked with.

When I started to identify and eliminate my tolerations and incompletes, I felt as if I transformed from a sponge to a powerful person—instead of allowing the negative energy around me to soak into me, it started to bounce off of me. I began to have more energy to take control of what I **could** control and change it for the better. Once you start identifying your energy sappers, you are putting yourself in the driver's seat of your own life.

As you list your various energy sappers, remember not to judge them, worry about them, or feel overwhelmed by them. By simply getting them down on paper, you're starting to confront them.

You may wonder why this step is necessary. You just want to drop a few pounds—why should you spend time jotting down the fact that your relationship with your overcritical father-in-law drives you nuts? Remember, everything in your life is related, and it all passes through you. Energy sapped from one place can affect every other part of your life.

Just becoming aware of your energy sappers and articulating them will bring them to the forefront of your mind. This is an amazing process. Just recognizing energy sappers can begin the process of eliminating, fixing, or resolving them. If that happens, go with it. But if it doesn't, that's fine. Don't get stuck on them. For now, getting them down on paper is great.

Once you get all your energy sappers out of your head and into your notebook, it is as if one of the cluttered blackboards in your brain has been erased. With a clean slate, you're ready to move forward.

Be aware that there is a delicate balance between confronting issues and creating problems for yourself. If you focus on small issues, you can magnify them and make the obstacle bigger and bigger. Rather, we are confronting obstacles to create opportunities for change and forward movement.

Finally, keep this great quote in mind:

> I've missed more than nine thousand shots in my career.
> I've lost almost three hundred games. Twenty-six times I've been
> trusted to take the game-winning shot and missed. I've failed over
> and over and over again in my life. And that is why I succeed.
>
> —Michael Jordan

Handling Challenges

Here are six tips to help you handle the challenges that come along as you journey toward balance:

1. **Use your gut as your guide.** Often we look to someone or something external to guide us through life's bigger challenges. Tap in to your own power, and use your gut (*not* your head) as your guide. Sure, you can use your knowledge, but try not to overthink or overanalyze anything. Your gut is an amazing guide.

2. **Turn to your support team.** Reach out to your supporters as you confront your obstacles. Your support team may have advice or may help you open your mind to strategies that may work for you. Even when your supporters don't have answers, they can listen. You know what real support means—you defined it in Chapter 5.

3. **Flip your focus.** It's normal to focus on problems, but it's not very helpful. Instead, try to flip your focus to what you *can* control and what you *can* do for yourself or others. If you know of a family in need of food, for example, make a meal, dessert, or gift basket for them. And if you don't have time to cook the meal, make a basket with all the ingredients. This will help take the focus off the stress in your life and fill you with good spirit.

4. **Stop trying to solve the problem.** When you focus really hard on solving a problem, you magnify it to the point that it's all you can think about. Paradoxically, sometimes the more you think about a problem, the harder it is to solve. Instead of fixating on what's wrong, shift your focus to all the good things going on in your life. For example, if you feel desperate to lose weight, try to put aside thoughts about calories and pounds and instead delve into something completely different and wonderful—reconnecting with friends, doing a favorite activity, volunteering to help others, and using your unique gifts to make a difference in the world. When you get totally wrapped up in living your life, your problems often take care of themselves.

5. **Let your vision propel you forward.** When no clear answer is presenting itself, go back to basics—your vision, your faith, and your core values. Think about your vision for your life, and let God guide you. If you lose your job, you can react by frantically applying for every job under the sun, whether you're really interested in it or not. Or you can spend some time really thinking about your vision for a happy, satisfied life. What are you doing in that vision? How are you spending your days? Once you have a really good sense of your vision, it will help guide your next steps in a calm, mindful way.

6. **Believe that somehow this will teach you something.**
    Almost every problem, difficulty, and negative experience has
    hidden lessons that help you benefit and grow—eventually.
    Believing that there's a lesson in every challenge helps make
    the challenge a bit easier to bear. Go back to other tough
    times in your life and look at the knowledge you gained from
    them. Then, have faith that you will someday learn from what
    you're coping with today. Trust that no matter how hard a prob-
    lem is, you will grow from having faced it.

Handling an Unexpected Twist

I love the whole process of putting up our Christmas tree—pulling
out the ornaments we've collected over the years, watching the kids
jumping around us, fighting over who gets to hang the decorations
and where things should go.

Putting up the tree itself takes about ten minutes. There are three
parts that snap together, and the white lights are pre-strung. So
that's the simple part—usually. A couple years ago, our basement
flooded, and when we put the tree together the following Christmas, we realized none of the lights worked. Michael tried everything, but there was no saving the lights. The wiring was all rotted
from the inside.

Back in the basement, my hubby found a set of colored lights and
did a quick wrap-around to see if we liked them. Of course, LuLu and
the Little Man were all in favor of colored lights! Lu said, "Mommy,
those lights are *WAAAAAYYYYY* better than the other ones we had
last year!" The lights did have a magic to them—they were a little
larger and had a nice glow.

So, the hubby said, "What do we do? Do I just string them over the top? The old lights are strung between every branch." My little smile made my husband cringe—he knew this quick fix wasn't the answer. Stringing the bright, hopeful colored lights over the broken ones didn't sit well with me. We needed to take the tree apart, remove the old lights, and replace them with new ones. Michael didn't love this idea. He even offered to run to Home Depot for another tree. But we both knew that wasn't the answer, as this tree was barely four years old. So, branch by knotted branch, we carefully removed every single light.

Lu and the Little Man cheered us on. They couldn't wait to hang the ornaments. The anticipation was priceless. Still, it was definitely an exercise in patience. I silently repeated a word that helps me in situations like this: *aretae*, which means "patience is a virtue." When my husband would breathe an extra-loud huff, I reminded him how beautiful the tree would look when we finished. As we worked, I pondered the message that the tree was giving us: a message of authenticity, change, hard work, patience, and ultimately, after almost four hours spent removing the lights, appreciation.

The tree decorating lasted throughout the day. When we finished, we took a step back in awe of the beautiful tree that had almost made us rip our hair out. Michael and I agreed it was so worth it.

Confronting Replacement Behaviors

I used to be a big-time stress-eater, especially when I was in my yo-yo dieting phase. I would follow whatever diet du jour I happened to be on, but then something would happen—a bad day at work, a stressful situation, an emotional meltdown—and all of a sudden I would run for the cabinets and go off my diet! I would beat myself up and feel discouraged, and then wait for a better time to start again.

Why did these problems cause me to eat?

As I mentioned earlier, diets treat symptoms. Typically there is a UHO, a root issue, challenge, or obstacle. And sometimes, eating is a response to an emotion. I call this a replacement behavior. When something is missing from one area of our lives, we often replace it with a negative behavior. Replacement behaviors happen all the time—you eat when you're stressed; you fight with your spouse because you're frustrated with your job; you shop for shoes because you break up with your boyfriend (okay, this may actually be a necessary behavior . . .).

Once you identify the reasons you overindulge, you can make a conscious decision to choose another, healthy replacement behavior and essentially retrain your response.

When I realized I ate as a response to stress, I decided to replace my stress-eating with something much more productive: getting organized. I even went so far as to hang a sign on my refrigerator that said, *Stress = Organize,* and another on my cabinets that said, *Food = Fuel,* to remind myself that I should eat to energize and not to emote. To this day, if my husband comes home and he sees me going haywire organizing paperwork or closets or whatever, he asks me, "What happened?" He knows organizing is now my stress response.

Just recently, my husband went to the doctor because he had some back pain. The doctor did a few tests that raised a concern, which immediately sent my husband for a CT scan of his abdomen and pelvis to rule out pancreatic cancer and renal disorders. We were shocked—this came out of left field. My husband thought he had pulled a muscle. During the weeks of testing and waiting, I became worried and stressed. I knew I had to be strong, focusing only on each step of the process and not going down the what-if path. But during weak moments, I would give in and Google a word I saw on a test result, try to play doctor (which I definitely *do not* recommend), and get a little freaked out. During one of those days, I found myself heading straight for the kitchen cabinet. As I opened the door, it hit me. I was about to stress-eat. I wasn't hungry at all.

I stopped myself and grabbed a box of Christmas cards. Instead of printing out address labels to make the task go more quickly, I busied myself in carefully handwriting addresses. I made a rule that I would not be sloppy or rushed. I would take the time to focus on the beautiful task of spreading joy (and of course sharing a photo of my LuLu and Little Man) to friends and relatives around the country.

Michael came into the kitchen and saw me at the table with my Christmas card station all set up. He smiled, knowing it was my

NOTE FROM AN INSPIRISTA
Denise

I've realized that totally getting rid of stress is impossible for me, but I often find myself eating in response to stress. Mindless eating when I'm stressed is a huge habit of mine that happens often and, most of the time, without me even realizing until after the food is in my mouth. I know it needs to be replaced by a healthier habit, an alternative to mindless eating. The first thing that came to mind was doing my nails. I thought, "Hey, why not give it a try?" But doing my nails was a difficult thing to commit to, since I am constantly using my hands, so I thought, "Why not just one nail?" I could do that, and I could still do whatever chore I was doing and let the one nail dry. It was an interesting experiment. I realized I had a lot of stressful moments, because even one nail at a time, as the day went on, all of my ten nails were pretty and painted. With this alternative habit, I was able to eat healthy, and I was more aware of how much stress I have in a day. I think this is going to be my new response to stress.

Denise

response to the stress of waiting for his test results. "Babe, you are so funny," he said. We both laughed, and I shed a couple of tears too.

Later that week we received good news, putting our minds at ease. I am so glad I didn't eat myself into a coma, as I would have done in the past, because that wouldn't have done us any good. Choosing to do the Christmas cards made me feel a bit joyful and definitely in appreciation of this gift of life. (Although my sister-in-law told me a few days later that she received three Christmas cards from us—at least I spread triple the joy to her!)

To determine your unhealthy behaviors, be brutally honest with yourself. Take a no-excuses attitude and get to know yourself even better.

1. Identify emotions that trigger unhealthy behaviors. Are you overeating or skipping workouts because of boredom, anger, depression, or frustration? Or to avoid communicating with someone?

2. Figure out healthier replacement behaviors. For example, organize, call a friend, go for a walk, meditate, write in your B.A.L.A.N.C.E. Journal, visualize your favorite vacation spot, vacuum, take your dog for a run, pray, or listen to loud music.

3. Set up a retraining, or reminder, system so you can retrain that trigger!

B.A.L.A.N.C.E. Tip

Ditch the Stretch Pants

Don't wear clothes that grow with you. Being comfortable is important, but growable clothes often hide the feeling of fullness that can definitely lead to indigestion and feeling terrible later. You want to enjoy the meal before, during, and after. So *no* stretch pants.

Coping with Common Obstacles

We have to embrace obstacles to
reach the next stage of joy.

—Goldie Hawn

By understanding the obstacles that can tangle you on your balance journey, you can prepare yourself and be ready when they come your way. Here are some of the most common obstacles as well as tips on confronting them.

Obstacle: Expensive food

Take charge: When you're trying to eat healthy food, money can sometimes be an obstacle. Here are some things you can do to overcome it:

- Coupons for fresh food aren't often readily available, but you can find them online. Google the exact foods you'd like to buy (i.e., *coupons fresh strawberries*) and you will find discounts and coupons that will help lower the cost.

- Go frozen or canned to save big time. Frozen veggies such as spinach or broccoli and fruits such as strawberries and blueberries are way cheaper than fresh produce. Many are frozen or canned immediately after harvesting, so they have the same nutritional value as fresh produce. When buying canned or frozen fruits or vegetables, be sure to choose those without any added sugar or salt.

- Stock up on sale foods. When produce is on sale, buy extra and freeze it.

- Go beyond the supermarket. Look for bargains at farmers

markets, alternative grocers such as Trader Joe's, food co-ops, community gardens, and local farm stands.

- Make a grocery list with your budget in mind, and stick to it. The extras that we toss in the shopping cart really add up!

- Make beans a staple in your diet. Kidney beans, black beans, white beans, pinto beans, baked beans—they're full of vitamins and fiber and are cheap, cheap, cheap. Buy them in cans or save even more money choosing dried beans that you cook up yourself.

Obstacle: Fear

Take charge: I've had clients tell me they feel they've lost control and are completely imbalanced, but fear keeps them at status quo. If you want to move forward, believe in yourself, hold strong to your faith, and surrender fear. Fear can be debilitating because it blocks us from taking inspired risks. Kick fear to the curb by setting your intentions, taking actions, and reaching small goals. Achievements of any kind actually help build our confidence. So take that step forward, and if you happen to fall, pick yourself back up and keep on moving! There will be a lesson or a meaning somewhere down the road that will unfold when you are aware and in tune.

Obstacle: A crowded mind

Take charge: Meditate, even for a minute. Prayer is speaking to God, and meditation is listening. Your innate wisdom has so much to tell you, but you won't hear it unless you shut everything else out and listen. Even a *minute* of meditation goes a long way—certainly you can find a minute here and there to clear your mind. Close your eyes, breathe deeply, and let go of your fears. A clear mind helps us kick out the junk and connect with our purpose, so picture a white light and focus.

Obstacle: Unsupportive people

Take charge: It's frustrating when the people around you are not in line with your goals. When this happens, you usually can't change others, but you can control what *you* do, how *you* react, and *your* own actions. Focus on what you *can* do to move forward and still be the healthiest version of yourself possible. Don't give other people's negative behaviors any more power in your life—try to focus only on the things you can control.

Obstacle: Hurtful comments

A journalist once asked me if I had ever received hurtful comments from strangers about my weight. My answer was, "Who hasn't?" People had commented on my weight and size for as long as I can remember. In grammar school, when I was the tallest kid in the class, my nickname was Big T. When I grew up, strangers asked me when I was due, and I wasn't even pregnant. Once, when I was grocery shopping, a little boy asked me if he could rub my belly. His mother just laughed and said, "Never mind him. He thinks you're pregnant." To this day, almost daily I encounter someone commenting on my weight. Some say I'm thin, others think I'm not thin enough. It's actually quite funny—one day in a store, a cashier asked me how I stay so thin. Later that afternoon, a clothing store clerk told me, "We have great tops that will hide your waistline!" And I hadn't even changed my outfit.

Take charge: Thank goodness I don't take people's remarks seriously anymore. Now I just smile at them. It was not easy at first to turn my ears and heart off to people who obsess over body size—after all, it's everywhere. But once I learned to love and accept myself, my mind-set completely shifted. And as a matter of fact, I turned my heart *on* to those people, showing compassion to where they are in their own life journey and size obsession. Here are some things I learned about dealing with comments from people about weight and size:

- Practice self-care. Love and nurture yourself no matter what shape or size you are. Nourish your body, mind, and spirit while practicing self-care.

- Don't fire back—inquire. Being curious is always a good thing. Asking questions opens up your mind to what others are thinking. When people say something that doesn't feel right or kind to you, ask them about it. Don't be defensive or assume they mean the worst. Try simple questions, like, "What do you mean by that?" or "Why do you ask?" This allows them to explain what they actually mean—and if they spoke carelessly, to realize how hurtful comments can be. I'm sure we've all put our feet in our mouths at some point and would have loved the opportunity to explain, so give others that opportunity.

- Realize that sometimes it's just your interpretation. Haven't you ever read into something and realized later you were completely wrong? When our self-esteem is low, we tend to look for negative comments and assume everything is meant to hurt us. I distinctly remember being in the gym locker room watching girls laugh and totally assuming they were laughing at *me*. I felt awful all day, until I later learned they were laughing at a comment scratched into the locker! Remember, if you look for negativity, you will always find it, even if it doesn't truly exist.

- Be kind. It can feel difficult not to immediately get offended or hurt. But by staying strong, you won't allow other people's stress or negativity into your heart. Open up to the human being—they have their own story that may explain their behavior. Be compassionate. Instead of being defensive, you'll feel positive energy inside you. Energy is contagious, so why not pass along your positive energy? Kindness inspires people.

Tart but Sweet

Years ago, whenever I had a problem, I would stew on it forever. I'd call up every one of my friends, ask for advice, vent, circle back and forth, and seesaw up and down trying to figure out the answers. The problem would take hostage of my brain, and it was all I could think about until there was some sort of resolution or so much time had passed that the problem faded into the background of my mind.

I can't imagine how many hours I wasted. I was so wrapped up in my own world—it was just a tangled mess. As I got a little older, and the problems got a little tougher, somewhere, somehow over the last decade, I learned a profound lesson:

> When life hands you lemons,
> make *someone else* lemonade.

Whether it's volunteering with Enchanted Makeovers, helping a friend organize her office, or paying for a stranger's cup of coffee— just connecting with the world around me in a positive way can almost immediately lift my spirit. Honestly, I can't remember exactly when or how this dawned on me, but truly when I realized I should step outside of myself, help others, and stop wasting time on empty worrying, my whole world changed. And just by virtue of experience, it became a lesson.

The sun seemed a bit brighter. The clouds became more beautiful. The rain, which once symbolized despair, turned into a blessing, a cleansing, soulful dance. Of course, I am human. And there are times when I have to vent with tears or talking, but where I once took forever to get over problems, now it takes just moments.

And although I am writing about it, the proof is in the action. This is something that words really can't teach and money can't buy. We find ourselves in other people; we find our unique gifts when we have nothing else left but those to use.

> The most beautiful people we have known are those who have known defeat, known suffering, known struggle, known loss, and have found their way out of the depths. These persons have an appreciation, a sensitivity, and an understanding of life that fills them with compassion, gentleness, and a deep loving concern. Beautiful people do not just happen.
>
> —Elisabeth Kübler-Ross

Everyday B.A.L.A.N.C.E. Technique: *Connect*

Stressful moments have a way of popping up when you least expect them. But having a list of tried-and-true Everyday B.A.L.A.N.C.E. Techniques can help you push away the frazzles and feel better quickly. One of my favorites is connecting. Sharing a moment of connection with another living being can tame your temper, pull down your defenses, distract you from your troubles, and replace distress with reassurance.

The connection can take many forms. You can connect with a family member, a friend, a coworker, a member of your support team, a mentor, or a neighbor. You can have a go-to connection such as your best friend or your spouse, or you can pick someone different depending on what's stressing you out. Discussing your troubles with someone who's been down the same path can be very encouraging.

Even an empathetic stranger can provide that pick-me-up human connection that warms your heart. Alice found her blood boiling at a large discount store's self-checkout line when she realized the customer in front of her was paying for a large order with dollar bills that had to be fed into the cash collector one at a time. After several minutes spent watching the woman fumble tediously with crumpled bills and wondering why she didn't pick the full-serve line, Alice glanced at another customer who rolled her eyes and smiled. That simple empathetic connection turned the moment from frustrating to silly, and she was able to relax and appreciate the goofiness of the situation rather than get steamed up with stress. And after all, everyone has a story, and the woman with the crumpled bills is no exception.

Connecting doesn't have to mean spending a lot of time with another person, although that's great if you can manage it. Even a quick phone call or a brief chat can make a big difference.

You can also connect with a pet. Anyone who owns a beloved dog or cat knows how comforting it can be to spend time together walking, playing, petting, or just sitting. My sister-in-law, Carol, cherishes her dog, Flurry; the adorable Dalmatian is a source of pure joy for her and her family! Dogs in particular can lend such a calming presence that they're sometimes paired up with children undergoing scary tests in hospitals and with lonely nursing home residents. Studies show that petting a dog can lower blood pressure, improve mood, and generate feelings of well-being. I'm sure a purring cat can have the same effect when curled up on someone's lap.

When you connect with another living thing, whether a human or an animal, you're reminded of the fact that you're not alone in the world. It helps put your stressors in perspective.

INSPIRISTA INSIGHT
Power of Community

In this very busy, fast-paced, plugged-in world, it's easy to get caught up in the hustle and bustle of life and forget the incredible gift of connecting off-line and right in our communities.

As a child, joining a club happens regularly—I remember being a Girl Scout (and I am so proud of my little Lu, who is now a Daisy herself!) and being in the chorus. We even had a club in high school for poets and writers. As an adult, joining a club may seem frivolous at first, but on the contrary, being a part of a club, organization, or community often enriches our lives and fills our spiritual tanks.

Joining a community is amazing for so many reasons: sharing interests, such as scrapbooking, swimming, writing, or reading great books; having a supportive group of people who share your goals, hopes, faith, and dreams; and working together for a greater good in volunteering, reaching out, or sharing your gifts with the world. And sometimes being part of a group is exactly what we need to just play, let loose, have fun, and tap in to our inner child. So give yourself permission to just go with it and get involved.

Summing Up

In this chapter, we worked on defining the obstacles that prevent you from meeting your goals, discovering unidentified hidden obstacles, and brainstorming ways to surmount your obstacles. We also discussed ways to confront problems at their source rather than using unhealthy eating to cope with their symptoms, and we looked at methods to confront some of the most common obstacles that come up as you seek a life of balance. Finally, we reflected on the value of connecting with others to reduce stress and generate calmness.

In the next chapter, we'll talk about engaging—committing completely to changing your life for the better, living passionately, and learning from failure.

. . . .

Chapter Eight

E is for
Engage and *Experience*

You cannot help but learn more as you take the world
into your hands. Take it up reverently, for it is an old
piece of clay, with millions of thumbprints on it.

—John Updike

. . . .

My husband and I feel as if LuLu and Little Man have been in our lives forever. We can hardly remember a time without them, and we are blessed to have them in our world. We have learned so much from them in the past six years. They are the loves of our lives.

Looking at the world through their eyes has been an incredible gift. It's allowed us to see some of the moments that we adults often miss. Using a child's perspective can allow us to engage in the world around us in a way that allows our hearts to open up and more fully experience the gift of life.

We are born in awe, constantly amazed at the world, inspired by nature, and fearless. It's a beautiful way to live, and unfortunately it's a perspective many people lose over the years. Imagine regaining that childlike point of view and reconnecting with that part of yourself. It sounds impossible, but it's not. We really can add that essence back into our grown-up life view.

Seeing the world in an awe-filled, inspired, fearless way—engaging fully and completely in the world around you—is the topic of the last step of the B.A.L.A.N.C.E. Program. In this chapter, we'll focus on engaging.

You've come so far since the beginning of the program. You analyzed your relationship to food, diets, and the worries and concerns of your life. You let go of the baggage that has held you down and added in choices and behaviors that will help you feel balanced and whole. You created a renewed life vision, learned to set goals, and gathered a set of tools that will allow you to navigate your balance journey and confront obstacles that pop up along the way. Now it's time to engage yourself fully in the life you envisioned by making a complete commitment to incorporating everything you've learned and discovered into your life. You've learned all the tools and techniques—now it's time to pull everything together and engage in a life of energy, passion, health, excitement, and happiness.

By now you know that I can't tell you exactly how to do this. The power to engage passionately in life has to come from deep within your soul. But I can give you plenty of guidance. You'll have 100 percent of my support. You'll also have a cheering squad of inspiring women who have completed the 30-Day Challenge online. They have offered to open their B.A.L.A.N.C.E. Journals and their hearts to you as real-life examples. Their thoughts, ideas, encouragement, challenges, and wisdom will help you create a life-engaging road map that you can depend on for years to come.

Engaging in Life

My mission in life is not merely to survive, but
to thrive; and to do so with some passion, some
compassion, some humor, and some style.

—Maya Angelou

What does engaging in your life mean to you? Here's what it means
to me:

Whatever you do, commit to it completely. Once you make a
choice that aligns with your vision and your core values, embrace
it 100 percent. Celebrate it. Enjoy it. Love it. Whether it's a small
choice (which soap to buy), a food choice (which breakfast to eat),
an exercise choice (which workout to do), or a major life decision
(which career path to follow), embrace it with energy and passion.
Even if it's a choice that doesn't align completely with your goals,
love it anyhow! If you have a deep-fried fish sandwich for lunch,
don't feel guilty about it—enjoy every bite. Savor the flavor, enjoy
the crunchy breading, luxuriate in the cool smoothness of the
tartar sauce, and appreciate the softness of the roll. If you're going
to eat it, love it.

Plug in to each moment. Engaging in life means plugging in,
feeling it, living it, being fully and completely awakened. Open
your eyes wider and engage in the world around you. Right now,
feel the paper of this book you are reading (or the case of the
electronic reader, if you've downloaded it), and feel the firmness
of your feet on the ground (or the softness of the couch you're
cuddled up on). Notice the temperature of the room, the light
pouring in the window, the taste of the water with lemon in
the glass by your side, the scent of the herb-encrusted chicken
you've got roasting in the oven. (Okay, you may not be roasting a

chicken, but we can dream, can't we?) Use all of your senses. The same goes for your emotions. Plug in to them, feel them, let them flow, and respond to them. If you are tired, plug in to rest. Allow yourself the comfort of closing your eyes, leaving your cell phone out of your bedroom, and allowing yourself to plug in—fully and without guilt—to sleep. (By the way, I know women who choose to remove all electronics from their bedroom, and they swear they sleep more soundly.)

Say good-bye to guilt. Nobody sticks perfectly to their goals. We all stray from our vision sometimes and make choices that don't line up. We are human; we don't always say or do the right thing. When that happens, don't get stuck in a cloud of guilt. Turn it into a positive experience by learning its lesson. Realize that your choices should make you feel alive and excited, not down and defeated. If you make an unhealthy choice, learn from it and then move forward. If you decide the giant pasta dish you had for dinner didn't fit into your day's goals, don't feel bad about it. Drink a tall glass of water, go for a walk, and spend a few minutes reviewing your goals so that next time you can try to make a choice that better aligns with them. Don't beat yourself up. That pasta was a learning experience. Everything that teaches us more about ourselves is a positive thing, so absorb its lesson and move on.

Relish the simple joys of life. Let's face it—most days are pretty routine. You get up, work, do some laundry, make dinner, exercise, put your kids to bed. But if you are fully, passionately engaged in life, it's so much easier to relish the simple joys that come along so many times every day. When you're engaged, there can be joy in every detail, in even the most mundane tasks. Notice it, appreciate it, and celebrate it!

Embrace the notion of motion. Aim to live *in* motion rather than just existing and *going through* the motions of life. Being in motion doesn't mean to go-go-go at a frantic pace—do that, and you'll miss some of the best moments. It means being fully invested in every moment of the day. Whatever you do, do it with passion. Breathe in the morning air. Sing in the car. Converse deeply about everyday occurrences with your family, neighbors, and friends. Make a breakfast in bed for your spouse or loved ones. Give yourself a pedicure, or go get one (be sure to turn your cell phone off). Write in a journal, frame your favorite photos, sit in your car and enjoy a sunset, write a thank-you note to your favorite childhood friend or teacher. Do what makes your soul stir so you can live well with passion and energy!

Learn from failure. How many times have you tried something and not succeeded? Believe me, I am a living testament to the motto: if at first you don't succeed, try, try again! The beautiful thing about failure is that it has so much to teach. Turning failure into opportunity can be hard, so here are three tips that can help:

1. *Look back for understanding.* When you fail, you want to crawl in a hole and forget about it. But you can't move forward if you're cowering in a hole. Evaluate what happened—the good and the bad. Be honest with yourself. What was the lesson? What was the gift in the imperfection?

2. *Ask for feedback.* Sometimes you can't define or face the reasons for your failure. When that happens, ask a supporter to help you confront the truth, look at the whole picture, and learn valuable lessons.

3. *Go back to the source.* Sometimes we fail because we're chasing a goal that doesn't really line up with our vision and core values. When failure strikes, reevaluate your goals and values, and listen to your heart. You may discover the failure was a blessing in disguise and that you really should be following a different path.

> As we drive along this road called life,
> occasionally a gal will find herself a little lost.
> And when that happens, I guess she has to
> let go of the "coulda, shoulda, woulda,"
> buckle up and just keep going.
>
> —Carrie Bradshaw, *Sex and the City*

Appreciate emptiness. There are times when nothing is happening. Instead of feeling bored and disappointed, engage with the moment and appreciate all the beauty in the peacefulness. Think of it this way: When you have a cold, you feel miserable. You can't breathe through your nose, you're coughing so much your head hurts, your throat is sore, and you don't have an ounce of energy. You lie in bed dreaming about the moment when you'll feel better. But then when the cold goes away, you forget how crummy you felt, and your life begins again. When you're fully engaged in life, you appreciate that empty moments are empty not just because there's nothing exciting going on but also because there's nothing terrible happening, either. Enjoy that! Take a deep, clear breath and relish the fact that you feel healthy. Run down the street and appreciate that your legs work. Smell a flower and savor the fact that your nose is so beautifully designed that it can extract joyful scents from something you pull out of the ground. Look at life the way my friend's son did when he was in preschool: when she asked him how his day was, he smiled and told her it was a good day, "because nobody threw up."

Live every minute. Time going quickly is not a misconception. Don't blink—your life can pass you by if you don't really live it. Embrace life, and live it! Do the things you love to do and you will attract new people and experiences into your world. If you love nature, find places to go for hikes, spend some time outdoors every day, and appreciate nature wherever you see it, even if it's just in glimpses from the window of your car. If you are a writer, buy a journal, grab a pen, and start writing. Spend more time doing what you wish you were doing instead of just thinking about what you think you don't have time to do. Engage in life, make the most of every experience you have, and you will be (as the song goes) "simply irresistible!"

Face a Fear

> The most difficult thing is the decision to act,
> the rest is merely tenacity. The fears are paper tigers.
> You can do anything you decide to do.
>
> —Amelia Earhart

My husband surprised me with a new bike. It had been over fifteen years since I'd actually owned a bike, and I have to admit, although I really did want to ride, I was pretty scared. Would I fall off? Would I be able to brake? Turn? Avoid parked cars? Veer out into traffic? Would I be able to go downhill? Uphill?

I took a few minutes to introduce myself to the bike and rode it gingerly up and down my block on the sidewalk. My neighbor saw me and smiled. I felt like I was eight years old again, on my bike for the very first time—cautious, slow, using my feet to slow down.

The next morning I woke up ready to really face my fears and ride that bike on the road. Little Man had just woken up, Michael was drinking his morning coffee, and LuLu was still asleep. "I'll be right back, hon. I'm just going to ride up and down the street for five minutes. I want to get my bearings."

My husband laughed. Just the day before, he'd ridden by the beach for almost two hours. "Okay, babe," he said. "Have fun!"

I rode onto the street—it wasn't so bad. I picked up speed, and it felt kind of exhilarating. Then I biked around my neighborhood, the wind in my hair, the sun on my face. "Woo-hoo!" I actually shouted out *loud*. A lady walking her dog laughed, and I waved—with one hand off the handlebars!

A few blocks away from us, homes are set on the water. It's beautiful and serene, with very little traffic. I biked up and down, back and forth, smiling the entire time. It was over forty minutes, and I could have gone longer, but LuLu would be waking up soon and I wanted to give her a good morning kiss.

I walked in the door singing. How happy I was to have faced my fear! *What will you do today to face a fear?*

Zen Quickies

Ten Ways to Engage Instantly in Life

1. Play a game from your childhood—checkers, Scrabble, Operation, Twister.

2. Sing in your shower, car, yard, or office.

3. Have a good laugh.

4. Apologize—don't let bad feelings linger.

5. Accept an apology.

6. Have a good cry.

7. Take the day off and lounge in sweats all day.

8. Get dressed to the nines for no reason.

9. Walk a neighbor's dog.

10. Cash in all of your spare change and give it to someone who could use a little help.

Engage in What You Set Out to Do: Your 30-Day Challenge

I've worked with many women who, during our first meeting, say they want to be healthy, but their actions were telling a different story. Over the course of thirty days, I challenge them to make changes so they can align their thoughts with their actions. Now I'm going to give you that same challenge: to commit fully to what you want and to engage wholeheartedly in what you're setting out to do.

But first, I want to share some comments from a few of the women who have participated recently in my B.A.L.A.N.C.E. Program.

> *I have had a weight problem all my life. Last year I started to work out at Curves, and I had been wanting to try Jennifer's class. Well, I did! In thirty days, I learned to be conscious of my eating, and now I feel better. I lost twelve pounds and have kept it off. I have tried lots of diets, and yes, I lose weight, but I always gain it back plus more! I guess your trainer/coach has a lot to do with it. Jennifer is very dedicated to what she is teaching and makes you feel very positive. She truly has helped my understanding that this is not a diet, this is the way people should eat to stay healthy.*

> —Susie, Curves Member and Challenge Participant

> *The past few weeks I feel so energized. And I feel wonderful knowing I made a great choice in my life to take Jennifer's B.A.L.A.N.C.E. Program. It was just what I needed to feel fabulous about myself!*

> —Melanie, Corporate Program Participant

> *When I first joined Jennifer's Curves, everyone was talking about her B.A.L.A.N.C.E. class. I was reluctant to try it because I*

heard it wasn't a diet. I made many excuses as to why it would maybe be unhealthy for me. I couldn't have been more wrong! Now I realize how healthy I can be without dieting! I regret not joining the class sooner. In thirty days, I am ten pounds lighter and much healthier! It helps to have Jennifer as such a motivating coach through it all. I hope to stay as determined as I am. Thanks, Jen!

—Marie, Curves Member and Challenge Participant

I took Jennifer's workshop two months ago, and now I've lost over twenty pounds. I feel very inspired. Overall, I have enjoyed my experience with Jennifer. I will continue to stay focused. Jennifer's class was so positive and motivating, and I learned more in six weeks than I have in my entire life!

—Jeanine, Workshop Participant

I have high cholesterol and osteoporosis but am reluctant to take medication. My friend suggested Jennifer's program as an alternative. I can honestly say I feel better, and I've lost weight too! My thanks to Jennifer, who encouraged me to overcome my fear of change. Her guidance has taught me to nurture my body and soul.

—Joan, Workshop Participant

Jennifer's program is a life-altering experience. Before taking her workshop, I never exercised or thought about my health. I didn't want to. Now my life has changed. Jennifer gave me the power and the know-how to want to take care of myself.

—Elaine, Workshop Participant

Having had a weight problem most of my life, I have tried every diet there is. None of them work! Jennifer's B.A.L.A.N.C.E. Program explains that you don't have to starve or deprive yourself of anything. This is a way of life, and it works. Trust me. I lost over forty pounds last year and have kept the weight off.

—Jennifer, Coaching Client and Curves Member

With Jen's coaching, I have been so successful, and I will keep going. I lost nine pounds in thirty days, and I have been losing since, but more importantly, I feel great. I love challenging myself to try new foods I might never have tried, and boy, they are delicious! Thanks, Jennifer, for opening my eyes and stomach to new wonderful things.

—Tina, Workshop Participant

I have done every diet imaginable—Weight Watchers, Atkins, Jenny Craig, you name it. I even had a gastric bypass. I always did them well, but I never felt like I actually learned anything or changed. So when I went off of them, the weight came back quickly. I joined your class, and have realized for the first time in my life, I'm not "doing a diet," I am actually discovering myself! I feel real changes in my thoughts and my actions. I am learning new behaviors! And, on top of all that, in just eight weeks, I've lost twenty-six pounds! Thank you for allowing me to be part of your B.A.L.A.N.C.E. challenge.

—Denise, Workshop Participant

Jennifer, since working with you, not only have I felt healthier and happier than ever, but I have also become way more open, tolerant, and patient. No other program has ever made me feel that way. Usually it's quite the opposite. A couple of years ago when I was redoing my kitchen, I went to a discount store and became so infuriated so quickly, I left and spent tons of money somewhere else. Now I am redoing my bathroom and decided to try the discount store again. My new, more-patient self stayed at *the store, and because of you, I saved over $10,000! So not only do you help people lose weight, you saved me money!*

—Clarice, Coaching Client

TAKE ACTION

. . . .

WHAT'S *YOUR* CHALLENGE?

Over the next thirty days, create a challenge for yourself. Push yourself outside of your comfort zone, try something new, enroll in a class, get involved in an activity, use your gifts, create new recipes, have some fun, light up a room, walk a little faster, or park a little farther away. Let your vision guide you, and remember, the possibilities are limitless.

You can choose a daily challenge, like some of these my clients have done:

- I got in touch with my younger self and started a jigsaw puzzle during the storm.

- I jumped rope for twenty-five minutes—I broke out into a sweat unlike I've felt in years!

- I walked three miles outdoors with some old friends.

- I packed all my meals for the week in Tupperware, and they look delicious.

- I donated my time in a soup kitchen. It was much healthier and far more fulfilling than being home, bored, and eating on the couch.

- I made a video of myself talking about what I wanted for my life, and I am even contemplating starting a blog about it. Maybe that will be tomorrow's challenge, definitely out of my comfort zone!

Or it can be a monthly challenge:

- I registered for three cooking classes at a county college to think outside the box!

- I joined a support group for women whose husbands are overseas.

- I began bike riding again, and I am choosing to eat only fresh, natural foods. I also joined Curves because having the support of other women is very helpful to me.

- I chose to be more pleasant at work and nicer to my coworkers. Believe it or not, I actually began a midday walking group with five other women in the office.

- I dusted off my art supplies and am going to begin painting again. This will get me out of my after-work rut of chips and dip before dinner.

- I am training for a thirty-mile walk to raise money for breast cancer.

Now you've got some ideas. How will you challenge yourself to change this month? What actions can you take to engage in what you set out to do? Join our online community of women and share your 30-Day Challenge with them!

. . . .

Making Engaging Effortless

Lately I've been really watching the birds fly, a lot. This morning I happened to catch a glimpse of one gliding just a few feet in front of me, and I marveled at the way it seemed effortless and carefree. Many people equate flying or soaring with success, but I think it's more than that; I also equate it with trust, faith, peace, and overcoming challenges.

When a bird flaps its wings, air is pushed down. This opposition in force lifts the bird in the air. It's not easy to oppose something. Baby birds have to trust that the flapping will take them in the air. They fall, they must get back into the air, and they fall again—they must have faith in themselves that they can fly. They must believe.

Once the bird hits the air, watching it fly is peaceful. I closed my eyes after I saw the bird this morning. I imagined the smooth feeling of flight, and I began to picture all the people that make difficult work seem effortless: A-Rod hitting a home run, Fred Astaire and Ginger Rogers dancing, Carrie Underwood belting out high notes. Effortless.

And this makes me think about life. *Can life really be effortless?*

Engaging in life may feel like it is going to take a lot of effort. You've already got a long to-do list, and now we are adding in challenges and new activities. I'm not going to lie—it does take work. But once you do the work, it becomes part of you.

Effortlessness does not mean without work or challenges. To me, living effortlessly means living with joy and lightness, releasing the weight on your shoulders, working hard but with a purpose, and living with passion. Oh yes, life can be effortless.

How do you define effortless? When does your life feel effortless? What work will you do to create what you want for your life? What ways can you begin engaging in life? My life feels effortless when:

- I breathe deeply.

- I am fully in the moment, connected to the present.

- I trust completely that everything happens for a reason.

- I witness my kids' pure joy over the little things—bubbles in the backyard, the sound of a motorcycle or truck rattling down the road, and seeing the neighbor when she's out walking her dogs.

- I choose faith over fear.

- I am grateful—not just back-of-the-mind grateful but truly steeped in gratitude and appreciation.

- I communicate my thoughts clearly, and I listen openly to others.

- I include fun and play in my daily life.

- I clear my mental plate and simplify, simplify, simplify.

- I turn the radio up loud and sing along with my favorite songs.

- I follow the flow of good energy.

- I step outside of myself and give to others.

Everyday B.A.L.A.N.C.E. Technique:
Experience

How we spend our days, is, of course,
how we spend our lives.

—Annie Dillard

The last Everyday B.A.L.A.N.C.E. Technique is all about creating an experience. When you're stressed, tired, harried, and just need a Zen Quickie, this final technique is amazing. It doesn't have to take long to have a profound impact on your mood and stress level. In just a few moments, with a bit of creativity, some imagination, and a sense of fun, you can bring about near-magical transformations. Think about it: all you need is a little glue, some glitter, a few sequins, and a couple rhinestones to turn an old pair of shoes into a pair of ruby slippers that can take you anywhere.

Start looking for ways to infuse everyday experiences with joy and happiness. Here are some suggestions for simple transformations:

Turn a shower into a spa treatment. Pick a soap that smells fantastic, and really take note of the scent. Breathe deeply in the shower. Be present. Don't let your mind wander to your to-do list—enjoy it with all of your senses.

You can also use some of your favorite kitchen ingredients to make a homemade scrub or hair treatment. Create a milk and honey scrub by mixing ⅓ cup sea salt, 1 tablespoon milk, a squeeze of honey, and a drop of olive oil. If your hair needs some

TLC, try this coconut hair treatment: add some coconut oil and a splash of coconut milk to your favorite conditioner. Or make your own conditioner by mixing coconut oil, coconut milk, an egg, and a teaspoon of honey.

Add meaning to your morning coffee. I love my morning coffee, so taking this ordinary activity to extraordinary is super-simple for me. I love using meaningful mugs. I'm not talking about fine china, but something that evokes a feeling or a memory—a dragonfly mug that reminds me of my grandmother, for example. And a mug decorated by my kids reminds me of how beautiful life is in a child's eyes. Be sure to switch it up so it doesn't become the same old mug.

Another way to make ordinary morning coffee an extraordinary experience is by creating simple versions of café-style coffee. Heat up some milk, froth it up with a whisk, add a dash of cinnamon, and turn your everyday coffee into café au lait. For a richer café-style blend, try a dark-roasted bean, such as French roast or Sumatra roast. Something rich in flavor will really jazz up your morning coffee. Having a few varieties of coffee on hand is a good way to keep it interesting—dark roast one day, hazelnut the next, and Colombian the following day.

Add pleasure to every encounter. We see people all the time—in the neighborhood, while walking the dog, and at school, the bank, toll booths, and stores. Instead of giving a nod or a wave, make every connection extraordinary. Smile, say hello, stop and chat. Smile with your eyes and be genuinely happy to see others. If you spread happiness to them, and they spread happiness to the next person they see, an ordinary activity can become a chain of joy.

Brighten someone's day. Recently, a complete stranger made my day. While I was at the convenience store, the woman in line beside me gave me a huge grin and said she liked my shoes! I immediately smiled back and complimented her on her handbag. These are little things, but they made us both smile. It made me think about how many simple ways there are for us to do something nice for each other. Here are just a few:

- At work, stick a note to someone's computer: *Great presentation at the meeting yesterday.* Or, *Thanks for always being there.* Or, *Love the necklace!*

- Give someone a sincere, unexpected compliment.

- Ask to see photos of someone's kids, new boyfriend, family, vacation, home, or whatever it is they love.

- Send a handwritten note for no reason at all to your spouse, children, mom, or best friend. Because they see you regularly, they will be extra surprised by this simple gesture!

- Follow up on previous conversations. Ask your colleague how her son is doing in his new college, whether your neighbor's new granddaughter has a new tooth, how your hairdresser's mother is feeling after her hip replacement surgery. People like to share, but sometimes they feel it's boring or selfish to talk about themselves unless they are asked. Remembering and asking about what's going on in people's lives can really brighten their day.

- Take off the shades, turn off the cell phone, and make eye contact with strangers.

- Give a small gift to someone who's been feeling down. Bake cookies, buy a bar of scented soap, or pick up a candle or a picture frame at a discount store. Wrap it in pretty tissue with a bow, enclose a short note, and let the person know you're thinking of her and are there for her if she needs help.

Write a love letter. There's something about writing out our feelings that is inspiring, cathartic, and connects us on a deeper level. Take a few minutes to write a love letter to anyone—your partner, your best friend, your mom, your dad, your children, your first influential school teacher, your neighbor who waters your plants, or your postal carrier.

Let the recipient know why you appreciate him or her. Use details. For example, if you love that your husband cleaned the car, write something like, *A fresh car, and you make me smile. I love you. XOX.* Or if your mom picked up your kids from dance class, try something like, *Ballet is beautiful and so are you. I love you. Thanks for always helping out.* Then mail the letter. Putting it in an envelope, sealing it, and stamping it give a little extra love-letter pizzazz to your note.

Move, move, move! If you want to live with passion and energy, being active is key. Exercise is important, of course, but so is living actively between workouts. Movement energizes you and ignites passion in all parts of your life. Here are simple things you can do anytime, even if you are not in your gym clothes or anywhere near a gym:

- Breathe deeply.
- Hold your tummy tight.
- Stretch your arms out wide.
- Do some side bends.
- Lunge up the staircase.
- Do calf raises while waiting in line.
- Don't drive through: actually park and walk.
- Offer to help carry something (a neighbor's groceries, a coworker's bags, or boxes that need to be moved).
- Twist and punch to whittle the waist and move those arms.
- Follow the next-level rule: push your activity up a notch by standing instead of sitting, walking instead of standing, running instead of walking.

Experience Life by Adding Sparkle to Your Soul

My mother always taught me that a little lip gloss goes a long way. Taking just a minute extra for some self-care can really make a difference in the way you feel. And although she was a licensed cosmetologist, Mom also taught me that real beauty cannot come from expensive makeup, a new hairstyle, or designer clothing. It comes from within.

I do like makeup—it's fun to play with and can change your look and sometimes your mood. I'm always amazed at how a swipe of lip gloss can add sparkle to your face. But I've also learned that there are many ways to add sparkle to your soul too. Smiling at a stranger, noticing the color of the leaves, dancing with your kids—these are things that make your soul smile, sparkle, shine.

We all have a light inside of us. Sometimes it's shining strong; other times we need to reignite our spark for life. Here are some soul sparklers for you—along with one last assignment for you at the very end of the list:

To Sparkle Every Day

- Smile. Be compassionate in all human interactions.

- Show public appreciation. Praise someone in front of family or coworkers, on a blog, or in some other public way.

- Write a joy list of your ten favorite things.

To Sparkle in Your Community

- Volunteer at your local shelter, soup kitchen, or senior center. Get to know the people inside and connect with them by listening and sharing stories.

- Clean up the park, the streets, or any place that needs some TLC. Dive in and beautify your community.

- Be a good neighbor by watering lawns, helping to remove snow, or stopping by with a pot of hot homemade soup on a cold winter day.

- Connect with children. Be a coach or umpire, color with a neighbor's toddler, offer to babysit, hold a newborn baby, or visit a children's hospital. Nothing makes the soul sparkle like experiencing the world through the eyes of a child.

- Vote in local elections, go to town meetings, and contribute your special gifts and unique talents to enrich your community.

- Share your stuff—the lawn mower, a bike, your car—there are always times when a neighbor could use some help but may feel awkward asking.

- Create community events: potluck suppers, picnics, horse and buggy rides, caroling, or open-house mixers with tea and cookies.

- Spread good news about neighbors' new grandchildren, promotions, and business ventures.

- Connect in your online community as well. Contribute or comment to blogs you read, or reach out to an old friend on Facebook with a happy memory or a random note.

To Add Sparkle to Your Body

- What you eat affects everything you do, think, see, and feel. It affects your productivity, attitude, relationships, and mood. Eat real food and feel real good; eat junk and feel like junk.

- Take two minutes in the morning and two minutes in the evening just to breathe.

- Get down! Doing yoga poses such as a downward dog, upward-facing dog, or hero pose for a couple of minutes a day is a great way to stretch your muscles, improve flexibility, and clear your mind.

- Get some sleep. Help yourself sleep better by not eating anything at least three hours before bedtime and preparing your body to relax. If your mind won't let you rest and keeps spinning with whatever has given you the blues, instead of counting sheep, count your blessings.

- Warm your sheets before bed. Soft sheets, just out of the dryer make for a cozy night and happier mornings.

- Move, move, move, and move some more!

- Get a massage. If your budget is tight, check out massage therapy schools that offer extremely discounted rates (or even free massages).

- Practice gratitude regularly. Give thanks even during difficult times. Gratitude relieves stress and tension in the body and makes your soul sparkle.

To Sparkle at Home

- Circles suggest harmony and unity, so make sure you have circles, such as wreaths, on your front door and inside your home.

- Once you've read a book, write a note in the cover about your thoughts on it, your favorite part, something personal. Create a book-giveaway basket, and every time someone enters your home, invite them to pick a book at random without looking inside. Whatever they choose will be the message they are meant to receive.

- Rid energy drainers: fill holes, fix squeaks, and replace bulbs and batteries for a clean, updated look.

To Sparkle at Work

- Write a morning to-do list. Bonus points for smiling when writing it.

- Organize your space bit by bit. Start by organizing just the space you're working in right now.

- Unsubscribe from every junk mail e-mail list you are on.

- Contribute toward creating a positive, pleasant work environment. Do not participate in gossip sessions with coworkers, as they just create negativity all around.

- Take a dance break—yes, at work.

- Give someone a list of all they've done that you're grateful for. Take a few minutes to make a list of ten or twenty things a coworker or colleague has done that you appreciate.

To Sparkle Behind the Wheel

- Tune your radio to something that makes you smile, laugh, or just relax—upbeat or soothing music, a book on tape, or your favorite talk radio show.

- Use your drive time to reconnect and fully experience the present moment.

- Send prayers and peaceful thoughts to crazy drivers. Don't get caught up in their road rage.

- Post your favorite quote or affirmation somewhere in your car.

- Silence your phone, especially on short trips. Not only will this create a more peaceful drive, but you won't be tempted to check it every time it dings or buzzes. Nothing is so urgent that it's worth risking your life or the lives of others on the road. Or create special ring tones for expected/emergency calls.

- Take a random drive to the beach, the mountains, or a park and watch the sun set or rise.

To Sparkle While Shopping

- Let someone with just one item skip ahead of you and your cart full of groceries at the checkout line.

- Ask the mother with her hands full if she needs help opening the car door.

- Put your shopping cart back where it belongs.

- If you see an item in the wrong section, return it to its proper place.

- Buy the person in line behind you at the drive-through a cup of coffee.

- Purchase something to donate—extra canned goods, toys, hats, or mittens. Or make something by hand and give it away.

Eat Sparkle-Worthy Breakfasts

- Cooked oat cereal with cinnamon

- High-fiber cereal with almond milk and fruit

- Egg-white omelet with salsa and low-fat cheese in a tortilla

- Egg-white omelet with cinnamon and maple syrup

- Toasted whole-wheat bread with a teaspoon of apple butter or peanut butter

- Toasted wheat English muffin with avocado and tomato

- Protein drink with fruit and wheat germ blended into a smoothie

- Plain low-fat yogurt with coconut extract and berries

- Pumpkin bran muffin with ½ teaspoon almond butter

Eat Sparkle-Worthy Lunches

- Chicken salad made with apples, celery, tarragon, lemon, and fennel tossed in a Dijon-yogurt dressing

- Tuna salad made with Dijon mustard and ½ teaspoon mayo on Wasa crackers

- Soup made with low-sodium broth, lots of veggies, and delicious herbs and seasonings

- Green leafy salad topped with chicken and tossed with olive oil and a splash of balsamic vinegar

- Veggie burger on toasted whole-wheat English muffin with marinara sauce

- Spinach leaves used as wraps for turkey, tomato, and hummus

- Fresh mozzarella, sun-dried tomato, and basil in a whole-grain pita

- Smoked salmon and cream cheese on Wasa crackers with tapenade

- Chili made with turkey or vegetarian, with beans, corn, celery, tomato, and onions

Eat Sparkle-Worthy Dinners

- Whole-grain pizza with fresh mozzarella, tomato, and basil

- Mediterranean chicken with tomato, olives, and white beans

- Broiled tilapia with rosemary and lemon served with couscous

- Chicken with lemon, olive oil, capers, and Dijon mustard, served with yams

- Wild salmon with fresh ginger and spices served over rosemary asparagus

- Vegetable stir-fry with olive oil and low-sodium soy sauce

- Grilled peanut shrimp made with natural peanut butter, fresh lime juice, cayenne pepper, and almond milk

- Chicken kebabs served with brown rice and grilled pears

- Seafood Crock-Pot paella made with tomatoes, scallops, tilapia, and veggies served over brown rice

TAKE ACTION

WHAT MAKES YOU SPARKLE?

Here's your final activity: write down five things that make your soul sparkle and share them with your online community. Have fun with it!

Acknowledgments

I have to thank so many people for being on this journey with me. I honestly feel every person I've ever known has contributed to the development of this book in some way, and many kind strangers, too!! I give the glory to God knowing that He has definitely been the source of the many random acts of kindness, the encouragement I've received, even the tests and trials (I know they have served many purposes), and for the miracle of working with such a phenomenal team of people to be able to deliver the message this book provides.

A huge thank you to my husband, my rock, my best friend, and our two precious gifts and my greatest teachers, Millana Elle and Ewing James—I know how blessed I am that you believe in me even more than I believe in myself. To my parents—words can't express the gratitude in my heart for always lifting me up and standing beside me no matter what. And Mommy, we've been through so much, so many fun escapades together!! Grandma Millie, I know you were up there helping and believing, too. I love you and miss you every day. To my mother-in-law, Ellie, thank you for everything, including watching the kiddies on Tuesdays so I could write and teach my classes! Danielle, Rich, Gail, Anthony, Carol, Joe—I don't know where I would be without your guidance, love, and support! You guys are amazing. To Katie, Michael, and Chris—I am so proud of each of you; you are such great role models for my munchkins, too!! And thank you Savannah for your smiles that melt my heart of course!

To my unbelievable literary team, thank you! Thank you! Thank you! Jumping for joy really *is* good exercise. Celeste—you believed in this book from the beginning; I am so fortunate to work with you! And you know you are more than an agent to me; you are truly a friend. Plus, thanks to you, I can say I know what it's like to be an athlete and have a whole bottle of Champagne dumped on my head! To the best collaborator in the world, Alice Kelly, what would I have done without you reining me in, keeping me focused, and sharing your knowledge and years of experience in writing books with me?! Thank you for dedicating yourself to this project. It was so much fun working with you on this book, and I miss our regular chats!! To my brilliant editor at Harper, Nancy Hancock, you can't imagine the impact working with you has had on my life. I have learned so much from you, and I am honored that you chose this book. Thank you for letting me "be me," listening, questioning, setting the bar high, and pushing me to reach it so we could provide a truly helpful tool, and always (beyond) lifting me up in your highest regard! Every writer needs a mentor like you—here's to happy, healthy, joyful women everywhere! And to the rest of the HarperOne team, including the "messengers" in helping the world know about my book, Suzanne, Claudia, Molly, Laina—your enthusiasm is a gift! I just have to pinch myself really. Thank you!

I have so much gratitude for the many teachers in my life, including Stephen Cluney, Dr. Dell, Dr. McGhee, David Harris Katz (remember, David, our conversation about field of dreams?!), and the late Carol Kiyak (Ms. Kiyak, you always encouraged my writing and I think of you often). And, Steve Cohen, WOW, my husband and I owe you and your wife an Italian dinner. Thank you doesn't feel like enough! I will never forget your kindness. Also, I would be remiss not to mention the courses I've taken at NYU, Spencer Institute, Wellcoaches, Life Coach Institute, Curves International, Monmouth University, and I also have learned so much in general from life, people, and experiences. . . . I know without these teachings this book would not have been written.

I am grateful to all of the people who support and love me "flaws and all," including my entire family, aunts, uncles, cousins, Mr. and Mrs. Vecchione, my dear friends Jessica, Jennie, and the Morrisys, my incredible assistant, Chris, my childhood girlfriends Jaime and Melissa, my Enchanted Makeovers family Terry, Ellen, Mary, and Marta, and many other phenomenal people who were once strangers who lifted me up in some way and are now ingrained in my heart, including Rob Longo, Rick, Donna, Joanne, Jacquelyn, Andrew, Amy, Rebecca, Barbara, Renee, and Carol . . . thank you!

Many thanks to Sue and Julie for introducing us to Curves and all your family did in 2001 to support our club opening, to the incredible people at Curves International—Becky and, of course, Gary and Diane Heavin—you have changed lives around the globe, including my family's, and I am eternally grateful. And to our entire Curves community, particularly Nancy, Connie, Kathy, Margie, Denise, Donna, Penny, Patti, Nancy, Amanda, Nathalie, Carolyn, Jenn, Georgia, Suzanne, Felicia, Michelle, Jess, Jennie—oh, what fun we've had together!! I want to also give special thanks to all of our dear members, my clients, and the participants who have joined in my "Challenge" classes over the years; I've learned so much from each and every one of you. Thank you for opening your hearts to learning from each other and exploring life together.

It is a gift to share my story thus far, the stories of some remarkable women I've had the pleasure of knowing, and the techniques I've discovered for finding and redefining balance. I know that if just one person sees themselves in me or any of the "inspiristas" featured in the book, then the words have done their work.